Genitourinary Ultrasound

Editor

LORENZO E. DERCHI

ULTRASOUND CLINICS

www.ultrasound.theclinics.com

Consulting Editor
VIKRAM DOGRA

October 2013 • Volume 8 • Number 4

ELSEVIER

1600 John F. Kennedy Boulevard • Suite 1800 • Philadelphia, Pennsylvania, 19103-2899

http://www.theclinics.com

ULTRASOUND CLINICS Volume 8, Number 4
October 2013 ISSN 1556-858X, ISBN-13: 978-0-323-22746-9

Editor: Donald Mumford

Ultrasound Clinics (ISSN 1556-858X) is published quarterly by W.B. Saunders, 360 Park Avenue South, New York, NY 10010-1710. Months of publication are January, April, July, and October. Business and editorial offices: 1600 John F. Kennedy Boulevard, Suite 1800, Philadelphia, Pennsylvania 19103-2899. Accounting and circulation offices: 6277 Sea Harbor Drive, Orlando, FL 32887-4800. Periodicals postage paid at New York, NY, and additional mailing offices. Subscription prices are $258 per year for (US individuals), $309 per year for (US institutions), $123 per year for (US students and residents), $289 per year for (Canadian individuals), $345 per year for (Canadian institutions), $308 per year for (international individuals), $345 per year for (international institutions), and $147 per year for (Canadian and foreign students/residents). To receive student/resident rate, orders must be accompanied by name of affiliated institution, date of term, and the signature of program/residency coordinator on institution letterhead. Orders will be billed at individual rate until proof of status is received. Foreign air speed delivery is included in all Clinics subscription prices. All prices are subject to change without notice. **POSTMASTER:** Send address changes to *Ultrasound Clinics,* Elsevier Health Sciences Division, Subscription Customer Service, 3251 Riverport Lane, Maryland Heights, MO 63043. **Customer Service (orders, claims, online, change of address): Telephone: 1-800-654-2452 (U.S. and Canada); 314-447-8871 (outside U.S. and Canada). Fax: 314-447-8029. E-mail: journalscustomerservice-usa@elsevier.com (for print support); journalsonlinesupport-usa@elsevier.com (for online support).**

Reprints: For copies of 100 or more, of articles in this publication, please contact the Commercial Reprints Department, Elsevier Inc., 360 Park Avenue South, New York, NY 10010-1710. Tel.: (+1) 212-633-3874; Fax: (+1) 212-633-3820; E-mail: reprints@elsevier.com.

Printed and bound by CPI Group (UK) Ltd, Croydon, CR0 4YY

Contributors

CONSULTING EDITOR

VIKRAM DOGRA, MD
Professor of Radiology, Urology, and
Biomedical Engineering, Director of Ultrasound
and Associate Chair for Education and
Research, Department of Imaging Sciences,
University of Rochester School of Medicine
and Dentistry, Rochester, New York

EDITOR

LORENZO E. DERCHI, MD
Professor and Chairman, Department of
Radiology, IRCCS Azienda Ospedaliera
Universitaria San Martino IST, University of
Genoa, Genoa, Italy

AUTHORS

MICHELE BERTOLOTTO, MD
Assistant Professor, Chief of Ultrasound,
Department of Radiology, University of Trieste,
Ospedale di Cattinara, Trieste, Italy

NANCY CARSON, MBA, RDMS, RVT
Department of Imaging Sciences, University of
Rochester Medical Center, Rochester,
New York

JEONG Y. CHO, MD
Department of Radiology, Institute of Radiation
Medicine, Clinical Research Institute, Seoul
National University College of Medicine, Seoul
National University Hospital, Seoul, Korea

CALOGERO CICERO, MD
Staff Member, Department of Radiology, San
Bassiano Hospital, Bassano del Grappa (VI),
Italy

FRANÇOIS CORNELIS, MD
Service d'Imagerie Diagnostique et
Interventionnelle de l'Adulte, Groupe
Hospitalier Pellegrin, CHU de Bordeaux,
Bordeaux Cedex, France

LIONEL COUZI, MD, PhD
Radiology Department, Université Bordeaux
Segalen; Nephrology Department, Service de
Néphrologie et Transplantation Rénale,
Groupe Hospitalier Pellegrin, CHU de
Bordeaux, Bordeaux Cedex, France

LORENZO E. DERCHI, MD
Professor and Chairman, Department of
Radiology, IRCCS Azienda Ospedaliera
Universitaria San Martino IST, University of
Genoa, Genoa, Italy

VIKRAM DOGRA, MD
Professor of Radiology, Urology, and
Biomedical Engineering, Director of Ultrasound
and Associate Chair of Education and
Research, Department of Imaging Sciences,
Faculty of Medicine, University of Rochester
School of Medicine, Rochester, New York

JEAN-LUC GENNISSON, PhD
Institut Langevin–Ondes et Images, ESPCI
ParisTech, CNRS UMR7587, INSERM U979,
ESPCI, Paris, France

NICOLAS GRENIER, MD
Service d'Imagerie Diagnostique et
Interventionnelle de l'Adulte, Groupe
Hospitalier Pellegrin, CHU de Bordeaux,
Bordeaux Cedex; Radiology Department,
Université Bordeaux Segalen, Bordeaux,
France

MARIANO IANNELLI, MD
Resident, Department of Radiology, Ospedale
di Cattinara, University of Trieste, Trieste, Italy

OUNALI S. JAFFER, MBBS, MRCP, FRCR
Research Fellow, Department of Radiology,
King's College London, King's College
Hospital, London, United Kingdom

HYEON H. KIM, MD
Department of Urology, Clinical Research
Institute, Seoul National University College of
Medicine, Seoul National University Hospital,
Seoul, Korea

SANG Y. KIM, MD
Department of Radiology, Institute of Radiation
Medicine, Clinical Research Institute, Seoul
National University College of Medicine, Seoul
National University Hospital, Seoul, Korea

SEUNG H. KIM, MD
Department of Radiology, Institute of Radiation
Medicine, Clinical Research Institute, Seoul
National University College of Medicine, Seoul
National University Hospital, Seoul, Korea

ERKAN KISMALI, MD
Staff Radiologist, Department of Radiology,
School of Medicine, University of Ege, Izmir,
Turkey

CHEOL KWAK, MD
Department of Urology, Clinical Research
Institute, Seoul National University College of
Medicine, Seoul National University Hospital,
Seoul, Korea

YANN LE BRAS, MD
Service d'Imagerie Diagnostique et
Interventionnelle de l'Adulte, Groupe
Hospitalier Pellegrin, CHU de Bordeaux,
Bordeaux Cedex, France

KYUNG C. MOON, MD
Department of Pathology, Clinical Research
Institute, Seoul National University College of
Medicine, Seoul National University Hospital,
Seoul, Korea

REFKY NICOLA, MS, DO
Department of Imaging Sciences, University of
Rochester Medical Center, Rochester,
New York

MEHMET RUHI ONUR, MD
Associate Professor of Radiology, Department
of Radiology, Faculty of Medicine, University of
Firat, Firat Universitesi Hastanesi, Elazig,
Turkey

PAUL S. SIDHU, BSc, MBBS, MRCP, FRCR
Professor of Imaging Sciences, Department of
Radiology, King's College London, King's
College Hospital, London, United Kingdom

ALCHIEDE SIMONATO, MD
Associate Professor of Urology, Department of
Urology, University of Genoa, IRCCS Azienda
Ospedaliera Universitaria San Martino IST,
Genoa, Italy

AHMET TUNCAY TURGUT, MD
Associate Professor of Radiology, Department
of Radiology, Ankara Training and Research
Hospital, Ankara, Turkey

MASSIMO VALENTINO, MD
Head of Radiology, Department of Radiology,
Ospedale di Tolmezzo, Tolmezzo (Udine), Italy

SADHNA VERMA, MD
Department of Radiology, University of
Cincinnati Medical Center, University of
Cincinnati, Cincinnati, Ohio

Contents

Preface   ix

Lorenzo E. Derchi

Contrast-Enhanced Ultrasonography of the Testes   509

Ounali S. Jaffer and Paul S. Sidhu

Contrast-enhanced ultrasonography of the testis can be readily performed, and provides crucial information regarding the underlying disease process not always apparent using conventional sonographic modalities. This supplementary information can be invaluable when deciding on appropriate management, potentially reducing the possibility of unnecessary orchidectomy. This article illustrates the technique of contrast-enhanced ultrasonography and reviews its application in both acute and nonacute testicular abnormalities.

Testicular Trauma: Role of Sonography   525

Refky Nicola, Nancy Carson, and Vikram Dogra

High-frequency ultrasonography is the modality of choice in the initial evaluation of patients with intratesticular and extratesticular trauma. Ultrasonography helps effectively triage patients for surgical and medical management. Testicular rupture is an important diagnosis that requires immediate surgical intervention to salvage the testis.

The Acute Scrotum   531

Lorenzo E. Derchi, Michele Bertolotto, Massimo Valentino, and Alchiede Simonato

Clinical history and physical examination do not always allow a firm differential among the different possible cause of acute scrotum, and imaging is needed to provide a diagnosis. Differentiating torsion from infection is a clinical emergency. Inflammatory conditions of the scrotum are the most frequent cause of acute scrotal pain in the adult population. The acute scrotum has several less common causes. This article outlines the ultrasonographic and Doppler findings in patients with acute scrotum of nontraumatic origin.

Postvasectomy Complications   545

Sadhna Verma

This article describes the anatomic changes following vasectomy, details potential complications following vasectomy, and illustrates the role of imaging in the evaluation of postvasectomy complications. This information is of value to diagnostic radiologists in determining whether a particular ultrasound finding is expected in a patient who has undergone recent vasectomy.

Ultrasound Elastography of the Kidney   551

Nicolas Grenier, Jean-Luc Gennisson, François Cornelis, Yann Le Bras, and Lionel Couzi

Ultrasound elastography is a new imaging tool under development that provides information about tissue stiffness. Well developed in liver diseases, its place is still preliminary in management of renal parenchymal diseases. This article reviews existing ultrasound elastography techniques and main results of the literature.

Contents

Elastography is a new tool under development and therefore application of ultrasound elastography to renal diseases requires further evaluation and validation before use in clinical practice.

Ultrasound Evaluation of Renal Masses: Gray-scale, Doppler, and More 565

Seung H. Kim, Jeong Y. Cho, Sang Y. Kim, Kyung C. Moon, Cheol Kwak, and Hyeon H. Kim

Ultrasound (US) is commonly the first step in the imaging evaluation of renal masses. Its main role is detection and characterization. Usually computed tomography or magnetic resonance imaging is needed for further characterization if a renal mass appears to have solid parts. This article describes US evaluation of renal masses in detail, including gray-scale US, Doppler US, and others.

Renal Masses as Characterized by Ultrasound Contrast 581

Michele Bertolotto, Lorenzo E. Derchi, Calogero Cicero, and Mariano Iannelli

Contrast-enhanced ultrasound (CEUS) depicts renal perfusion abnormalities and can assess vascularity of renal lesions. This article reviews the role of CEUS in the evaluation of renal masses, with a focus on differential diagnosis between cysts, solid tumors, and pseudolesions; characterization of complex cysts; and evaluation of lesions with equivocal enhancement at computed tomography. CEUS has an increasing role for the follow-up of patients undergoing tumor ablation. Emerging perspectives on monitoring angiosuppressive therapies in advanced renal cancer and intraoperative applications are discussed. Microbubbles can be injected without regard for renal function. Serious reactions are rarely reported, compared with iodinated contrast material.

Vascular Complications of Renal Transplant 593

Mehmet Ruhi Onur and Vikram Dogra

Renal transplant provides much longer survival than hemodialysis and peritoneal dialysis for patients with end-stage kidney disease. The prevention of complications in recipients improves survival rates. Imaging studies are crucial for early recognition of vascular complications of renal transplant. Ultrasound is the key imaging method in the evaluation of renal transplants in the immediate postoperative period and the long-term follow-up. Color flow Doppler ultrasound depicts most vascular complications.

Prostate Biopsies and Controversies 605

Ahmet Tuncay Turgut, Erkan Kismali, and Vikram Dogra

Transrectal ultrasound (TRUS)-guided biopsy of the prostate, the gold standard for the diagnosis of prostate cancer, plays a crucial role in the management of the disease. The absolute indications for performing a TRUS-guided prostate biopsy are abnormal digital rectal examination, elevated serum total prostate-specific antigen levels, and/or suspicious finding on TRUS examination. The procedure has several inherent shortcomings, including the risk of inadequate sampling of the gland. There are controversies about various aspects of the procedure, such as indications, preprocedural evaluation, sampling technique, that are explored throughout the article in light of the literature data.

Index 617

ULTRASOUND CLINICS

FORTHCOMING ISSUES

January 2014
Oncologic Ultrasound
Vikram Dogra, MD, *Editor*

April 2014
Emergency Ultrasound
Michael Blaivas, MD and Srikar Adhikari, MD, *Editors*

RECENT ISSUES

July 2013
Pediatric Ultrasound
Harriet J. Paltiel, MD, *Editor*

April 2013
Interventional Ultrasound
David L. Waldman, MD, PhD, *Editor*

January 2013
Obstetric Ultrasound
Eva K. Pressman, MD, *Editor*

RELATED INTEREST

November 2012, Volume 50, Issue 6
Radiology Clinics of North America
Male Pelvic Imaging
Kartik S. Jhaveri, MD, and Mukesh G. Harisinghani, MD, *Editors*

PROGRAM OBJECTIVE

The goal of the *Ultrasound Clinics* is to keep practicing radiologists and radiology residents up to date with current clinical practice in ultrasound by providing timely articles reviewing the state of the art in patient care.

TARGET AUDIENCE

Practicing radiologists, radiology residents and other healthcare professionals who provide care based on radiologic findings.

LEARNING OBJECTIVES

Upon completion of this activity, participants will be able to:
1. Review ultrasound elastography of the kidney.
2. Discuss ultrasound evaluation of renal masses.
3. Recognize renal masses as characterized by ultrasound contrast.

ACCREDITATION

The Elsevier Office of Continuing Medical Education (EOCME) is accredited by the Accreditation Council for Continuing Medical Education (ACCME) to provide continuing medical education for physicians.

The EOCME designates this enduringmaterial for a maximum of 15 *AMA PRA Category 1 Credit*(s)™. Physicians should claim only the credit commensurate with the extent of their participation in the activity.

All other health care professionals requesting continuing education credit for this enduring material will be issued a certificate of participation.

DISCLOSURE OF CONFLICTS OF INTEREST

The EOCME assesses conflict of interest with its instructors, faculty, planners, and other individuals who are in a position to control the content of CME activities. All relevant conflicts of interest that are identified are thoroughly vetted by EOCME for fair balance, scientific objectivity, and patient care recommendations. EOCME is committed to providing its learners with CME activities that promote improvements or quality in healthcare and not a specific proprietary business or a commercial interest.

The planning committee, staff, authors and editors listed below have identified no financial relationships or relationships to products or devices they or their spouse/life partner have with commercial interest related to the content of this CME activity:

Michele Bertolotto, MD; Nancy Carson, MBA, RDMS, RVT; Mahendra Kumar Chandran; Jeong Y. Cho, MD; Calogero Cicero, MD; François Cornelis, MD; Lionel Couzi, MD, PhD; Lorenzo E. Derchi, MD; James Donovan, MD; Nicolas Grenier, MD; Brynne Hunter; Mariano Iannelli, MD; Ounali S. Jaffer, MBBS, MRCP, FRCR; Hyeon H. Kim, MD; Sang Y. Kim, MD; Seung Hyup Kim, MD; Erkan Kismali, MD; Cheol Kwak, MD; Sandy Lavery; Yann Le Bras, MD; Jill McNair; Kyung C. Moon, MD; Donald Mumford; Refky Nicola, MS, DO; Mehmet R. Onur, MD; Lindsay Parnell; Paul S. Sidhu, BSc, MBBS, MRCP, FRCR; Alchiede Simonato, MD; Ahmet Tuncay Turgut, MD; Massimo Valentino, MD; Sadhna Verma, MD.

The planning committee, staff, authors and editors listed below have identified financial relationships or relationships to products or devices they or their spouse/life partner have with commercial interest related to the content of this CME activity:

Vikram Dogra, MD is editor of Journal of Clinical Imaging Science.
Jean-Luc Gennisson, PhD is a consultant/advisor and has royalties/patents for Supersonic Imagine.
Paul S. Sidhu, BSc, MBBS, MRCP, FRCR is on Speakers Bureau for Bracco SpA Milan, Hitachi, Inc. Tokyo, and Siemens AG Erlanger.

UNAPPROVED/OFF-LABEL USE DISCLOSURE

The EOCME requires CME faculty to disclose to the participants:
1. When products or procedures being discussed are off-label, unlabelled, experimental, and/or investigational (not US Food and Drug Administration (FDA) approved); and
2. Any limitations on the information presented, such as data that are preliminary or that represent ongoing research, interim analyses, and/or unsupported opinions. Faculty may discuss information about pharmaceutical agents that is outside of FDA-approved labelling. This information is intended solely for CME and is not intended to promote off-label use of these medications. If you have any questions, contact the medical affairs department of the manufacturer for the most recent prescribing information.

TO ENROLL

To enroll in the*Ultrasounds Clinic* Continuing Medical Education program, call customer service at 1-800-654-2452 or sign up online at http://www.theclinics.com/home/cme. The CME program is available to subscribers for an additional annual fee of USD 212.

METHOD OF PARTICIPATION

In order to claim credit, participants must complete the following:
1. Complete enrolment as indicated above.
2. Read the activity.
3. Complete the CME Test and Evaluation. Participants must achieve a score of 70% on the test. All CME Tests and Evaluations must be completed online.

CME INQUIRIES/SPECIAL NEEDS

For all CME inquiries or special needs, please contact elsevierCME@elsevier.com.

Preface

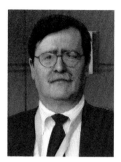

Lorenzo E. Derchi, MD
Editor

Ultrasonography can be considered the optimal initial investigation in a large variety of clinical problems regarding the genitourinary system. It is a noninvasive technique that has high diagnostic capabilities, is widely available, is portable at the bedside, and does not need the use of potentially nephrotoxic contrast media. In addition, with the use of high-resolution transducers, it can provide high-spatial resolution and high-sensitivity analysis of flow within superficial structures and organs. These characteristics make it a quite useful tool to evaluate the kidneys, especially in patients with renal impairment and, in the male patient, make it the preferred modality to evaluate the testis and to guide prostate biopsy. It is a relatively cheap technique that does not use ionizing radiation: then, considering ultrasound first is also the best approach in the era of cost containment and concern about the hazards of radiation exposure. Furthermore, even when not able to conclude the diagnostic workup of the patient, the results of an ultrasound examination can guide decisions about subsequent diagnostic procedures in the most appropriate way, thus rationalizing the patient's workup.

This issue of *Ultrasound Clinics* deals with ultrasonography in the evaluation of the kidneys and the testicles and as a guide to prostate biopsies. The authors must be commended for their contributions, since special attention has been paid to the role of recent technical advances in these fields, such as contrast-enhanced ultrasound and elastography. Although not still widely available, these techniques have significantly boosted the horizons of ultrasonography and have opened new perspectives, both in research and in clinical practice.We hope these articles will show the full potential of both "conventional" and "new" ultrasound techniques in the genitourinary system.

A special note of thanks must be given to Donald Mumford and the staff at Elsevier, who gave invaluable help to complete the issue.

Lorenzo E. Derchi, MD
Department of Radiology
University of Genoa
IRCCS Azienda Ospedaliera Universitaria San
Martino IST
Largo R. Benzi, 10
16132 Genova, Italy

E-mail address:
derchi@unige.it

Ultrasound Clin 8 (2013) ix
http://dx.doi.org/10.1016/j.cult.2013.08.003
1556-858X/13/$ – see front matter © 2013 Elsevier Inc. All rights reserved.

Contrast-Enhanced Ultrasonography of the Testes

Ounali S. Jaffer, MBBS, MRCP, FRCR*,
Paul S. Sidhu, BSc, MBBS, MRCP, FRCR

KEYWORDS

- Testis • Tumors • Infarction • Ultrasonography • Doppler ultrasonography • Microbubble contrast

KEY POINTS

- Conventional sonography of the testis has limitations, particularly regarding confidence in the nature of vascularity of a lesion.
- The addition of microbubble contrast aids the determination of the presence or absence of vascularity within a lesion.
- The presence of disordered vascularity on contrast-enhanced ultrasonography implies a malignant lesion, whereas absence of vascularity usually implies a benign lesion.
- Traumatic injury to the testis may be evaluated with contrast-enhanced sonography to detect viability of the testicular tissue and to direct surgery.
- Infarction and abscess formation in the presence of epididymo-orchitis is well defined on contrast-enhanced sonography.

INTRODUCTION

Ultrasonography remains the imaging investigation of choice for the evaluation of the scrotum because of its established accuracy, accessibility, low cost, and precise depiction of anatomy.[1] In most cases, sonographic assessment is the sole imaging technique required to achieve a diagnosis. While the sensitivity of B-mode ultrasonography in the detection of testicular masses nears 100%, it is not equivalent to a pathologic assessment.[2] Although some abnormalities such as testicular torsion and epididymo-orchitis will be supported by clinical history and investigations, sonographic differentiation of benign from malignant lesions is not always straightforward. Certain features may help narrow the differential, including location (intratesticular or extratesticular), lesion characteristics (solid or cystic), or vascularity detected on color Doppler ultrasonography (CDUS); however, in a

sizeable minority these features remain inadequate to determine the nature of the lesion.[3] In such cases, use of the full armamentarium of sonographic techniques, including contrast-enhanced ultrasonography (CEUS), should be considered.

CEUS is used widely in Europe and Asia and is established in cardiac and hepatic diseases, with applications in other organ systems, such as the testis, gaining wider recognition.[4] By determining vascular characteristics, uncertainty of diagnosis may be diminished with the management of patients altered, especially if there is clinical and imaging suspicion of benign etiology. The addition of CEUS allows the operator a greater degree of certainty, and facilitates a confident recommendation of "watchful waiting" or allows testes-sparing surgery to be undertaken.

CEUS has the added benefit of being simple to use, well tolerated, devoid of ionizing radiation, and performed in real time.[5] This immediate nature

Disclosure: P.S. Sidhu has received lecture fees from Bracco SpA, Milan.
Department of Radiology, King's College London, King's College Hospital, Denmark Hill, London SE5 9RS, UK
* Corresponding author.
E-mail address: ounali.jaffer@googlemail.com

Ultrasound Clin 8 (2013) 509–523
http://dx.doi.org/10.1016/j.cult.2013.06.003

of assessment can often alleviate undue patient anxiety encountered while awaiting further imaging investigations. This review describes the role of CEUS in the acute and nonacute scrotum, with particular reference to its clinical applications and limitations.

VASCULAR ANATOMY

Knowledge of the vascular arterial anatomy is desirable in fully understanding the pattern of contrast enhancement of the scrotum and its structures. The arterial supply to the scrotal sac and its contents arises from 3 sources: the testicular artery (arising from the aorta and supplying the testes); the cremasteric artery (a branch of the inferior epigastric artery, supplying the scrotal sac and the coverings of the spermatic cord); and the artery to the ductus deferens (arising from the superior vesical artery, which itself originates from the internal iliac artery). There are often multiple anastomoses between these 3 vessels, although the number and locations of anastomoses can vary between individuals.[6]

After piercing the tunica albuginea, the testicular artery branches into capsular arteries, which in turn branch into the centripetal arteries. These vessels course in the septations of the testicular parenchyma toward the mediastinum, where they further subdivide to form the recurrent rami. The recurrent rami branches then carry the blood away from the mediastinum into the testis. A recognized variant is the transmediastinal artery branch of the testicular artery, which persists in approximately 50% of patients.[7] It courses through the mediastinum to supply the capsular arteries, and is usually accompanied by a large vein. Knowledge of the defined vascular flow allows the operator to appreciate the directional flow of contrast in CEUS. During the arterial phase of imaging, the capsular and centripetal arteries are clearly demonstrated (**Fig. 1**), and distortion of this pattern should alert the operator to any underlying abnormalities.

ULTRASONOGRAPHY CONTRAST AGENTS AND IMAGING TECHNIQUES

Ultrasonography contrast agents consist of microbubbles, which are gas spheres of up to 10 μm in diameter, coated with a shell of different proteins, lipids, or polymers.[8] Microbubbles are comparable in size and mechanical properties with the erythrocyte and cross-capillary beds but do not pass into the interstitial space, making them true intravascular agents.[9] The coating of surfactant or polymer prevents rapid dissolving and

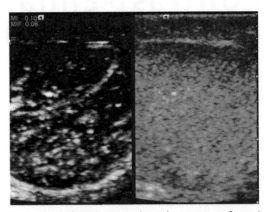

Fig. 1. Normal testis. Testicular enhancement after microbubble contrast administration, with vascular enhancement prominent in the larger vessels but with less enhancement in the testicular parenchyma.

agglomerating, as well as providing an inherent stability that enables recirculation to allow sufficient time for imaging, usually up to 7 minutes after injection.[10]

The gas core of the microbubble has a low density, which enables it to compress and expand in relation to the acoustic wave of alternating high and low pressures, resulting in emission of a strong echo. The microbubbles compress and expand in an uneven manner, causing asymmetric nonlinear bubble oscillation. Imaging techniques exploiting the nonlinear response of microbubbles are able to differentiate echoes arising from tissue from those arising from the microbubbles, suppressing signals from the background tissue. The two most commonly used specific contrast methods are pulse-inversion imaging and power modulation imaging. In the pulse-inversion method, 2 pulses are sent sequentially, with the second an inverted replica of the first. Both returning echoes are detected: the echoes from linear tissue produce no net signal, whereas the echoes from nonlinear reflectors such as microbubbles are asymmetric and are therefore detected, summated, and visualized.[11] In power modulation, 2 pulses identical in shape but with a 2-fold difference in amplitude are sent consecutively. On reception, the smaller pulse is rescaled by a factor of 2 and subtracted from the larger one. Again, with linear tissue this equates to zero signal, so the nonlinear microbubble signal remains and will be detected.[12] Microbubbles are known to reflect ultrasound waves at a very low Mechanical Index (MI), a property that is advantageous because it minimizes microbubble destruction. This low MI also reduces tissue harmonics and artifacts, and therefore facilitates the separation of tissue signal from that of the microbubble contrast agent.[4] In noncardiac practice in Europe, a sulfur hexafluoride gas with a phospholipid shell (SonoVue; Bracco SpA, Milan, Italy) is the agent used.[4] The shell component is metabolized by the liver and the gas is exhaled by the lungs. In general, this agent is safe with a low incidence of side effects, is not nephrotoxic, and does not interact with the thyroid gland.[5]

When applying microbubble contrast to testicular imaging, the normal examination procedure is followed; a high-frequency linear-array transducer is used, with the initial B-mode and color Doppler findings recorded. The standard practice is to administer the microbubble contrast intravenously via a cannula, followed by an immediate saline flush, targeting the focal lesion or the entire testis as required. The available microbubble agents work well when a transducer frequency of 3 MHz or less is used, the size of the microbubbles allowing the best resonance and subsequent detection at this frequency.[13] With higher frequencies ($\geq$10 MHz) the microbubbles do not resonate as efficiently, and a higher concentration of microbubbles (still within the dose allowed) is used.[14,15] Contrast dynamics can also vary because of differing blood volume content, method of supply, and flow dynamics. In the liver, the dual supply of hepatic artery and portal vein results in an arterial, portal, and late phase. In the testes, much like the kidney, there is an afferent arterial supply only. Because of differing vessel size and blood distribution in the testis, microbubble detection after injection is delayed and movement is slower. Whereas bubble detection in the liver and kidneys may occur within 10 to 20 seconds of injection, contrast detection within the testes is usually not seen before 20 seconds.[16] Initially the microbubbles are detected in the arteries, followed rapidly by parenchymal enhancement. Typically the scrotal wall will demonstrate lesser enhancement in comparison with the testis and epididymis. As there is no accumulation of microbubbles within the parenchyma of the testis, enhancement usually declines over a variable period of time, and often only minimal residual enhancement is evident 3 minutes after injection.

As the assessment of focal abnormalities during the arterial phase of imaging is usually critical, the optimization of imaging parameters must be performed before contrast enhancement. By setting MI at a minimum and placing the focus at the end of the field of view, microbubble destruction can be minimized. Gain should be set at a level so that background tissue echoes or noise artifacts are not present. It is recommended that gain modification should not occur while assessing the contrast-opacification characteristics of a lesion, so as to avoid ambiguity between true contrast enhancement and iatrogenic changes in intensity.[17] All examinations should be timed by use of the internal clock, and archived as single images and movie clips.

TESTICULAR TUMORS

Testicular carcinoma represents 1% of all neoplasms in men and is the most frequently encountered malignancy in the 15- to 35-year-old age group.[18] Patients typically present with a painless palpable scrotal mass or vague discomfort in the scrotum. Risk factors for the development of testicular carcinoma include: previous testicular tumor, family history, undescended testis, cryptorchidism, intersex syndromes, and infertility. Overall, prognosis is generally excellent, with survival rates at 10 years in excess of 95%.[18]

Most often, testicular tumors are of homogeneous low reflectivity in comparison with the surrounding testicular parenchyma; however, appearances can vary and include highly reflective heterogeneous lesions with solid, calcified, or cystic components.[19] B-mode ultrasonography is ideal for the detection of small lesions, with sensitivity approaching 100%; however, with specificity as low as 44%, definite differentiation of testicular cancer from benign scrotal masses is not always possible on B-mode alone.[2] CDUS imaging is routinely performed for evaluation of testicular lesions to demonstrate an increase in vascularity. Presence of increased or altered vascularity, although not specific for a diagnosis of malignancy, will aid the operator to better define the abnormality.[6] However, even after optimization of CDUS settings, vascularity may not be clearly established in small lesions (<1.5 cm).[4] This drawback is attributed to the technical limitations of Doppler imaging as opposed to a true absence of flow.[20] The principal advantage of CEUS is its ability to more clearly define vascularity, depicting minimal vascular flow in a dynamic manner, with accurate assessment of supplementary features such as preservation of vascular morphology, as well as "washout" characteristics of a lesion. If a benign vascular pattern is established, a more confident recommendation of monitoring with follow-up, as opposed to immediate surgery, may be advocated.[21]

There may be some differences in the vascularity seen in testicular tumors with CEUS. An understanding of the various types of testicular tumors is important.

Germ-Cell Tumors

Testicular germ-cell tumors are the most common type of testicular cancer, with a frequency of 90% to 95%.[22] Germ-cell tumors arise from spermatogenic cells and are divided into seminomatous and nonseminomatous types, a distinction that can determine prognosis. Tumor-marker assessment is important: α-fetoprotein (AFP) can be raised in yolk-sac tumors and teratomas, whereas human chorionic gonadotropin (hCG) may be raised in seminomas and choriocarcinoma.[23]

Seminoma

Seminoma is the most common pure germ-cell tumor, accounting for 35% to 50% of all germ-cell tumors, and is particularly radiosensitive.[24] In comparison with nonseminomatous tumors, it usually occurs in an older man with an average age at presentation of 40.5 years.[25] On B-mode sonography, seminomas typically appear as a solid, round, homogeneous low-reflectivity mass without calcification, although larger tumors may be heterogeneous and lobulated.[26] CDUS usually confirms the presence of hypervascularity, but accurate lesion interrogation can be restricted by the lesion size, as small lesions may incorrectly appear as avascular. Because of the superior spatial and temporal qualities of CEUS, real-time imaging of the microcirculation can be achieved, allowing resolution of flow within small tumors that cannot be imaged on color or power Doppler. As such, by demonstrating hyperenhancement within these tumors, including those smaller than 5 mm in diameter, CEUS is a more sensitive tool than CDUS.[21] Typically CEUS of seminomas will demonstrate a rapid enhancement in comparison with the surrounding parenchyma, with loss of the normal linear vascular pattern. Washout of microbubble contrast within the lesion is usually rapid, but with persistence of the abnormal "crossing" vessels within the lesion (**Fig. 2**).[27]

Nonseminomatous germ-cell tumors

Nonseminomatous germ-cell tumors (NSGCT) predominately occur in men aged in their 30s. Of all the subtypes, mixed germ-cell tumors (40%–60%) are the most frequently encountered in clinical practice.[28] Embryonal carcinoma is the most common component, and is often combined with teratoma, seminoma, or yolk-sac tumor.[25] Correspondingly, the tumor may demonstrate diverse ultrasonographic appearances dependent on the proportion of each component. Frequently, the tumors are of a heterogeneous echo-texture, but may also exhibit ill-defined margins, echogenic foci (hemorrhage, calcification, or fibrosis), or a cystic component (true cyst or necrosis).[6] Increased vascularity is not always a feature, and may lead to an inaccurate diagnosis of a benign lesion such as segmental infarction.[27] In such circumstances, CEUS could facilitate an accurate differentiation between a benign and malignant

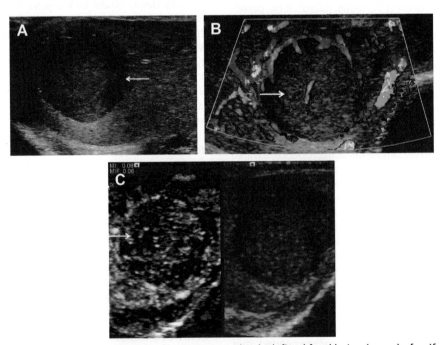

Fig. 2. Seminoma. (*A*) B-mode sonography demonstrates a clearly defined focal lesion (*arrow*) of uniform low reflectivity. (*B*) Color Doppler sonography demonstrates internal vascularity within the lesion (*arrow*). (*C*) Contrast-enhanced ultrasonography demonstrates early enhancement and rapid washout with abnormally configured vessels and pockets of nonenhancement (*arrow*) within the lesion.

entity. By virtue of the contrast agent being entirely intravascular, detected microbubble movement is always within vessels. As such, visualization of a haphazard pattern of microbubble movement within a lesion indicates abnormal vascularity and favors a malignant entity.[27]

Embryonal cell carcinoma, in its pure form, is the second most common single-histology tumor, but accounts for only 3% of all testicular malignancies; seminomas and mixed germ-cell tumors dominate.[29] Embryonal cell carcinoma typically occurs in younger men and tends to be more aggressive than seminomas, with tunica albuginea infiltration and distant metastases often identified at presentation.[25] These tumors are often heterogeneous and ill defined, and blend imperceptibly into the adjacent testicular parenchyma. In the authors' experience CEUS appearances can be variable, ranging from hypervascular lesions with increased enhancement in the early phase with rapid washout, to lesions with minimal but demonstrable enhancement (**Fig. 3**).

Choriocarcinoma is a rare tumor in its pure form (0.3%).[30] It carries the worst prognosis of any germ-cell tumor, with a high level of hCG usually correlating with a poor prognosis. Microscopic vascular invasion is common, with early hematogenous tumor dissemination to the lungs, liver, and brain.[30] Ultrasonography often demonstrates a heterogeneous solid mass with areas of hemorrhage, necrosis, and calcification. CEUS evaluation allows differentiation between the tumor tissue and hemorrhage, with increased enhancement during the arterial phase and early washout of the viable tumor, in comparison with nonenhancement of the hemorrhagic component.[14]

Yolk-sac tumors are the infantile form of embryonal cell carcinoma, and occur most frequently in children younger than 5 years.[31] The tumors are rare in adults except as a component of mixed germ-cell tumors. The sonographic features are nonspecific and similar to those of a mixed germ-cell tumor, with heterogeneity, cystic change, and areas of calcification on B-mode sonography. and haphazard microbubble movement within vessels on CEUS.[32–34]

Teratoma can be found in any age group. In children, it is the second most common testicular tumor and is often benign. In adults, the lesion is less frequently encountered (2%–3% of testicular neoplasms); however, unlike in children, tumors in the adult should always be treated as malignant.[6,28] The sonographic appearance of a teratoma can vary according to the differing composition of its germinal layers (endoderm, mesoderm, and ectoderm). As such, teratomas are often complex tumors with a heterogeneous echo-texture and cystic change. Echogenic foci

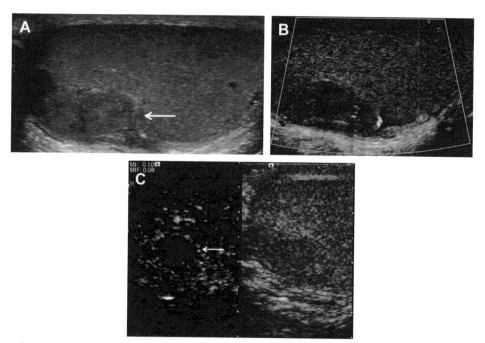

Fig. 3. Embryonal cell carcinoma. (*A*) A focal heterogeneous testicular abnormality is demonstrated on B-mode sonography (*arrow*). (*B*) No color Doppler signal is identified within the abnormality. (*C*) Following the administration of microbubble contrast, no contrast flow is seen within the center of the lesion, but enhancement in the periphery is present (*arrow*).

within the tumor may represent calcification, cartilage, or immature bone.

Sex Cord–Stromal Tumors

Sex cord–stromal tumors are the second most prevalent primary neoplasm (4%) after germ-cell tumors.[6] The lesions are typically small and are often detected incidentally, although painless testicular enlargement and gynecomastia (due to raised hormonal levels in 30%) are both recognized in this tumor type.[35] The majority (90%) of sex cord–stromal tumors are benign, with the 2 most common types being Leydig cell (derived from the sex cords) and Sertoli cell (derived from stroma).[27]

Leydig cell tumor is the most common sex cord tumor and can occur in any age group. Malignant Leydig cell tumor is a recognized, uncommon occurrence in the elderly.[6] The tumors typically appear as well-circumscribed homogeneous hypoechoic lesions on B-mode ultrasonography.[36] Larger tumors may exhibit some internal as well as peripheral hypervascularity on CDUS, but smaller lesions, which are the most commonly encountered in clinical practice, often appear devoid of flow.[37] CEUS is an invaluable aid in this often encountered diagnostic conundrum (**Fig. 4**). Typically the tumor will demonstrate

hyperenhancement in the arterial phase, but unlike in germ-cell tumors, the enhancement will persist with washout only evident in the delayed phase of imaging.[14,21] Clinical management can therefore be influenced, with less aggressive surgical options or follow-up being viable alternatives to orchidectomy.

Sertoli cell tumors are particularly rare (<1%) and, compared with Leydig cell tumors, are less likely to secrete hormones; the vast majority are benign.[38] The tumors can be divided into 3 histologic subtypes, namely sclerosing, large-call calcifying, and classic Sertoli cell tumors, with variable sonographic appearances according to the histologic subtype. Sertoli cell tumors are often well circumscribed, round, and lobulated, with calcification seen in the large-calcifying subtype. Vascularity may or may not be present on CDUS, with CEUS findings similar to those of Leydig cell tumors.

Mesenchymal Tumors

Mesenchymal tumors of the testis, both benign and malignant, are rare and include leiomyomas, neurofibromas, hemangiomas, and adenomatoid tumors (**Fig. 5**). Sarcomas include osteosarcoma, fibrosarcoma, rhabdomyosarcoma, leiomyosarcoma, and Kaposi sarcoma. The CEUS characteristics of these tumors are yet to be clearly defined.

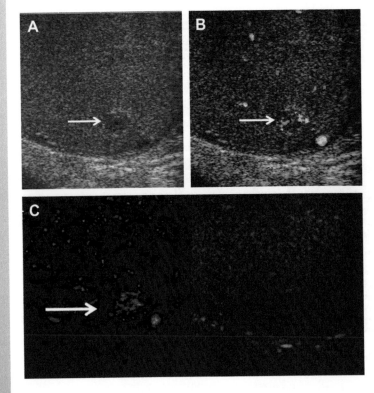

Fig. 4. Leydig cell tumor. (*A*) B-mode sonography demonstrates a small 4-mm hypoechoic lesion (*arrow*). (*B*) Color Doppler sonography identifies increased vascularity within the lesion (*arrow*). (*C*) Contrast-enhanced ultrasonography demonstrates early and persistent enhancement of the lesion (*arrow*), a characteristic that appears to differ from those of malignant tumors.

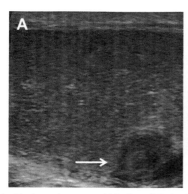
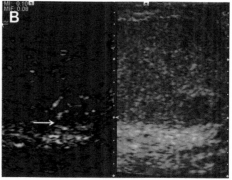

Fig. 5. Intratesticular adenomatoid lesion. (*A*) An 8-mm mixed-reflectivity lesion (*arrow*) is identified within the right testicle. (*B*) After microbubble contrast administration, there is enhancement (*arrow*) followed by early washout.

Lymphoma and Leukemia

Lymphoma can occur in the testis as a primary abnormality, as an initial manifestation of otherwise occult disease, or as the site of disease recurrence. The disease accounts for 5% of all testicular tumors, although testicular involvement occurs in less than 1% of patients with lymphoma.[39] Certain features such as age of occurrence (usually >60 years), bilateral involvement, and constitutional symptoms (25% of patients) can be useful clinical discriminators.[22] Almost all tumors are B-cell lymphomas, with diffuse large B-cell lymphoma the most common (80%–90% of cases).[40] Gray-scale sonography may show homogeneous hypoechoic testes, hypoechoic lesions of various sizes, or striated hypoechoic bands with parallel hyperechoic lines radiating peripherally from the mediastinum.[41] Infiltration of the epididymis (63%) and the spermatic cord (40%) are common.[42] On CDUS, testicular lymphoma always demonstrates hypervascularity.[43] With diffuse infiltration, differentiation from orchitis may be difficult; both entities show a similar pattern of hypervascularity, with vessels traversing in parallel.[44] Similar ambiguity can be found with CEUS, and differentiation from orchitis or seminomas is not always possible on imaging alone. As such, CEUS does not offer any useful supplementary information, as often the diagnosis of lymphoma is based on correlation with clinical findings (**Fig. 6**).

Although primary leukemia of the testis is rare, secondary involvement is common, with leukemic infiltration of the testis found in 40% to 60% of patients at autopsy.[6] Because of the blood-gonad barrier, chemotherapy agents cannot penetrate into the testis, conferring a poor prognosis and making the testis a prime location for extramedullary recurrence. The sonographic appearances are similar to those of lymphoma.[45]

Metastases to the testis are rare (<1%) and most commonly arise from a prostate or lung primary.[46]

Epidermoid Cysts

Epidermoid cysts are the commonest benign tumors of the testis, although they account for only 1% to 2% of all resected testicular masses.[47] Patients are usually between 20 and 40 years of age and typically present with a painless testicular mass. Four sonographic appearances have been described, with features varying according to the degree of maturation, compactness and quantity of keratin, and the quantity and distribution of calcium within the cyst[48]:

- Type 1: Classic "onion-ring" appearance with alternating hyperechoic and hypoechoic layers
- Type 2: Densely calcified mass with an echogenic rim
- Type 3: Cyst with a rim and either peripheral or central calcification
- Type 4: Mixed pattern, heterogeneous and poorly defined

Although the sonographic features of epidermoid cysts are characteristic, they are not pathognomonic. A critical distinction between epidermoid cysts and a malignant lesion is the absence of any vascular signal; an epidermoid cyst is a "true" cyst.[49] However, the absence of vascular signal may not negate operator uncertainty, as it is recognized that slow flow can escape color Doppler detection. CEUS is more sensitive for detecting vascularity and may increase operator confidence.[50] Patel and colleagues[20] demonstrated a lack of internal enhancement in all epidermoid cysts evaluated. Although peripheral rim enhancement was found in larger lesions, this phenomenon was attributed to an increased density of

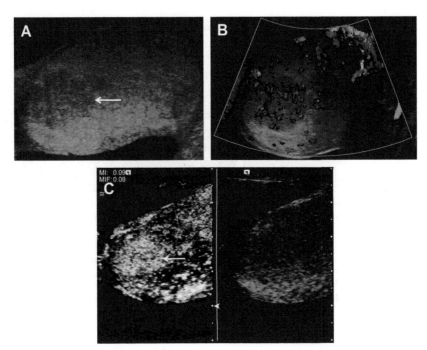

Fig. 6. Lymphoma. (*A*) B-mode sonography demonstrates a large low-reflectivity lesion within the testis (*arrow*), which infiltrates the epididymis in a 60-year-old man. (*B*) Color Doppler sonography confirms the lesion to be hypervascular. (*C*) Contrast-enhanced ultrasonography demonstrates early enhancement (*arrow*) and rapid washout.

vessels surrounding the lesion by virtue of a mass effect caused by compression of the normal testicular parenchyma; supported by a lack of such enhancement in smaller lesions. As such, the authors suggest that CEUS evaluation to confirm the absence of flow should be considered the hallmark in epidermoid cyst assessment (**Fig. 7**).

Cystic Lesions

The recognition of simple testicular cysts is normally straightforward, with an anechoic center surrounded by a thin imperceptible wall and a degree of posterior acoustic enhancement. Where there is wall irregularity or possible solid components, differentiation is more difficult. In the authors' experience, CEUS can demonstrate enhancement of the wall in cystic tumors and in lesions with vascularized internal solid components; this enables differentiation not only from simple cysts but also from cysts that contain internal nonenhancing debris (**Fig. 8**). Similarly, tubular ectasia, which represents benign dilatation of the tubules of the rete testis, can be evaluated by CEUS in unclear cases. Again, an absence of flow helps secure the diagnosis, with certainty increased if lesions are present in both testes and in those older than 50 years.[51]

ACUTE SCROTUM

Sonographic assessment of the scrotum can be invaluable in the acute setting, as the accurate differentiation of testicular torsion from epididymo-orchitis and other scrotal abnormalities is not always possible by physical examination alone.[52] The diagnosis of testicular torsion based solely on clinical examination can result in a false-positive rate of up to 50%, with consequential but unnecessary surgical exploration.[53] Studies have shown that the use of CEUS can achieve diagnosis in the acute scrotum when conventional B-mode and Doppler imaging remain inconclusive.[14,54,55]

Spermatic Cord Torsion

Spermatic cord torsion occurs following the twisting of the spermatic cord and interruption of the vascular supply to the testes. The condition is a surgical emergency because delayed diagnosis or misdiagnosis can be catastrophic, with irreversible ischemia detectable after 6 hours of testicular artery occlusion and complete infarction established by 24 hours.[56] Two types of testicular torsion are recognized: extravaginal and intravaginal. Extravaginal torsion is found in the newly born and is often asymptomatic. Intravaginal torsion is

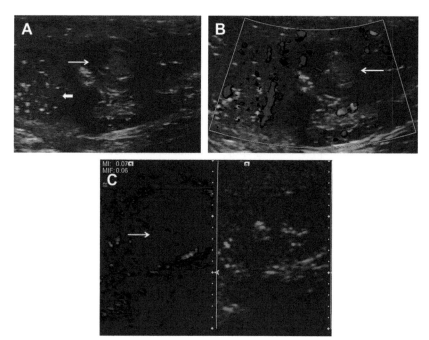

Fig. 7. Epidermoid cyst. (*A*) B-mode sonography demonstrates a well-circumscribed, solid, mixed-reflectivity lesion (*long arrow*) with identifiable "onion-skin" rims. Incidental note is made of testicular microlithiasis (*short arrow*). (*B*) Color Doppler sonography demonstrates an absence of flow within the lesion (*arrow*). (*C*) Contrast-enhanced ultrasonography confirms the findings with an absence of enhancement within the lesion (*arrow*).

typically associated with pain of sudden or insidious onset, nausea, and vomiting, and is frequently followed by swelling of the ipsilateral scrotum. A purported predisposing factor for intravaginal torsion is the "bell-clapper" deformity, whereby a narrow mesenteric attachment from the spermatic cord to testes allows the testes to fall forward within the cavity of the tunica vaginalis and rotate.[57]

The sonographic appearances of spermatic cord torsion begin with the development of venous

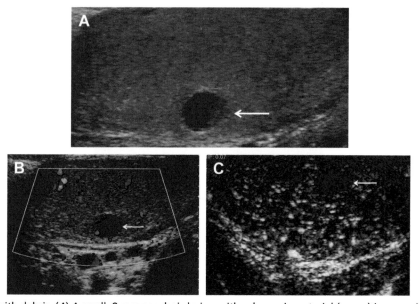

Fig. 8. Cyst with debris. (*A*) A small, 8-mm anechoic lesion with echogenic material (*arrow*) is seen within the testicle. (*B*) No internal color Doppler signal is demonstrated within the echogenic material located within the lower aspect of the cyst (*arrow*). (*C*) Contrast-enhanced ultrasonography demonstrates absence of enhancement of the echogenic component (*arrow*) and excludes the possibility of a cystic tumor.

congestion and subsequent edema, visualized on B-mode sonography by enlargement of the testis and decreased echogenicity. As the ischemia progresses, the testis appears heterogeneous and hypoechoic, and indicates infarction, whereas hyperechoic areas represent hemorrhage.[58] The epididymis becomes progressively larger and more heterogeneous, and it may be possible to identify the twisted spermatic cord, termed the "whirlpool" sign.[59] Color Doppler sonography can be used to differentiate between epididymo-orchitis, whereby there is increased vascularity, and torsion, with a reduced or absent blood supply.[60] It is imperative that settings are optimized to detect low-velocity flow, at the lowest repetition frequency and lowest threshold.[6] After this, vascularity of the testis can be assessed and should be compared with the asymptomatic side to serve as a baseline. At present, the use of CEUS for the detection of torsion has not been established.[4,55] There is agreement, however, that the ambiguity that may arise from the presence of artifacts when evaluating slow-flow Doppler can be avoided using CEUS.[14,55] Also, by avoiding the optimization process when evaluating Doppler flow, the

examination could potentially be conducted more rapidly (**Fig. 9**).[55]

There is potential that CEUS could be useful in the pediatric population, assessing for possible spermatic cord torsion. The absence of color Doppler signal in the pediatric patient could be misleading, as the poor sensitivity at detecting color flow in the smaller testis may lead to a false-positive diagnosis of torsion.[61] CEUS is not susceptible to artifacts, and should assist in the diagnosis of torsion by improving the sensitivity of flow detection. To date the safety of microbubble contrast in the pediatric population has not been established, and studies need to be performed in both the adult and pediatric populations to determine the clinical efficacy of evaluation of torsion using CEUS.

Segmental Testicular Infarction

Segmental testicular infarction is an infrequent finding in patients presenting with an acute scrotum.[62] Ultrasonography depicts a low-reflectivity or mixed-reflectivity area, which may be wedge-shaped or round.[63] Wedge-shaped areas with absent color Doppler signal can be

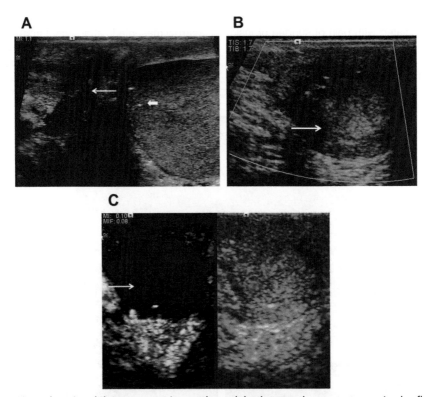

A

B

C

Fig. 9. Spermatic cord torsion. (*A*) A transverse image through both testes demonstrates a mixed-reflectivity, atrophic right testicle (*long arrow*), with microlithiasis (*short arrow*) identified within the normal-appearing left testicle. (*B*) Color Doppler sonography fails to demonstrate any discernible intratesticular vascular flow in the abnormal right testis (*arrow*). (*C*) Contrast-enhanced ultrasonography demonstrates a complete absence of vascularity throughout the testis (*arrow*) and confirms the diagnosis of a "missed" torsion.

attributable to benign segmental infarction with greater confidence than those that are more rounded in configuration: the concern with rounded lesions is true differentiation from a poorly vascularized tumor. CEUS allows for better characterization of such lesions in the subacute stage by clearly demarcating the avascular lobules and, in some cases, the perilesional rim enhancement.[64] Rim enhancement may be secondary to perilesional inflammatory changes or a mass effect (**Fig. 10**).

The chronologic evolution of segmental infarction can be depicted by CEUS. Often, within a month the perilesional enhancement disappears, the lesion decreases in size, and intralesional vascular "spots" appear within the abnormality.[64] As such, the combination of CEUS findings, change in size of the abnormality, and absence of raised tumor markers will often allay any concerns of a malignant process.

Venous Infarction and Intratesticular Abscess

Venous infarction and intratesticular abscess of the testis may occur in cases of severe epididymo-orchitis. The pathologic process is a continuum: initially, the swelling associated with epididymo-orchitis leads to occlusion of the venous drainage of part of or the entire testis, which culminates in infarction.[65,66] Eventually infarction leads to tissue breakdown and necrosis, with the subsequent development of an intratesticular abscess.[67]

Conventional imaging may not allow the confident differentiation of tumor or arterial infarction from venous infarction or abscess formation.[68] Lung and colleagues[16] showed that the differentiation of these entities may be possible by CEUS: a combination of a more rounded appearance, absence of intralesional enhancement and lesion location (central testis) favors the diagnosis of venous infarction or abscess. However, differentiation between venous infarction and abscess may not be possible on CEUS imaging alone, as both were found to have irregular borders, rim enhancement, and vascular projections (**Fig. 11**). In addition to epididymo-orchitis, venous infarction may occur in hypercoagulable states, whereas formation of intratesticular abscess can be secondary to mumps or trauma.[67]

Orchitis and Epididymo-Orchitis

Epididymitis is the most common cause of intrascrotal inflammation with the retrograde ascent of pathogens such as *Escherichia coli* and *Chlamydia trachomatis*, the usual route of infection. Secondary testicular inflammation caused by the direct spread of infection from the epididymis (epididymo-orchitis) occurs in 20% to 40% of cases; whereas isolated inflammation of the testis (orchitis) remains rare.[69] A combination of clinical (fever, leukocytosis) and imaging findings secure the diagnosis. Gray-scale sonography in isolation is

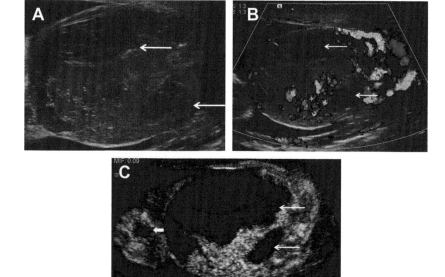

Fig. 10. Segmental testicular infarction. (*A*) There are 2 focal mixed-reflectivity abnormalities (*arrows*) identified on B-mode ultrasonography in a patient with clinical evidence of epididymo-orchitis. (*B*) No color Doppler signal is evident within either abnormality (*arrows*). (*C*) Contrast-enhanced ultrasonography clearly depicts the segmental areas of infarction (*long arrows*) and identifies a small epididymal abscess (*short arrow*).

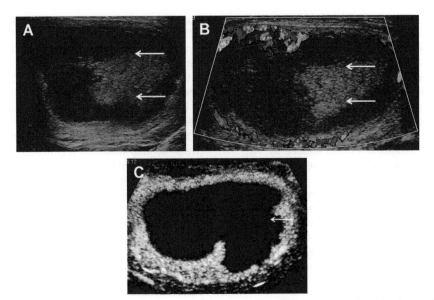

Fig. 11. Venous infarction of the testis. (*A*) B-mode ultrasonography demonstrates a focal testicular abnormality of mixed reflectivity (*arrows*). (*B*) No color Doppler signal is demonstrated within the lesion (*arrows*). (*C*) Contrast-enhanced ultrasonography demonstrates a marked differentiation between the normally enhancing parenchyma and the nonenhancing region of infarction (*arrow*).

normally nonspecific, with diagnosis often reliant on CDUS evaluation.[70] The demonstration of hyperemia within the epididymis, testis, or both on CDUS is considered the hallmark of scrotal inflammation. The detection of intratesticular venous flow greatly supports orchitis, as it is rarely seen in the normal testis. In uncomplicated infection CEUS adds little. However, as the presence of secondary complications such as hemorrhage, abscess formation, thrombosis of the spermatic cord, or venous infarction may introduce uncertainty, in such cases CEUS will clearly demonstrate nonenhancement of a central avascular component, and enhancement of peripheral rim and septa in abscesses, as well as an absence of flow within thrombosed spermatic vessels in cases of funiculitis.[4,14,16,55]

TESTICULAR TRAUMA

Testicular trauma is usually apparent from the clinical history, and occurs most frequently in men aged between 15 and 40 years. CEUS, by virtue of its exceptional demonstration of parenchymal vascularity, allows clear depiction of the extent of injury with fracture lines, tunica albuginea interruption, and scrotal hematoma, and the exact quantification of viable parenchyma more reliably assessed than on conventional sonography or CDUS.[55] CEUS allows the operator a more confident evaluation of 2 clinically important features: the presence of testicular rupture and the extent of viable testicular tissue (**Fig. 12**). Testicular rupture is considered a surgical emergency, as the preservation of testicular viability requires

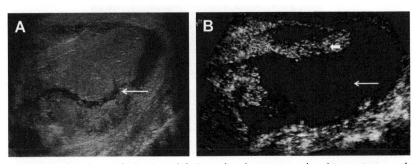

Fig. 12. Traumatic testicular devascularization. (*A*) B-mode ultrasonography demonstrates a heterogeneous "shattered" testis with a clearly demarcated fracture line (*arrow*). (*B*) On contrast-enhanced ultrasonography, there is clear differentiation of the viable testis (*short arrow*) from the remaining devascularized parenchyma (*long arrow*).

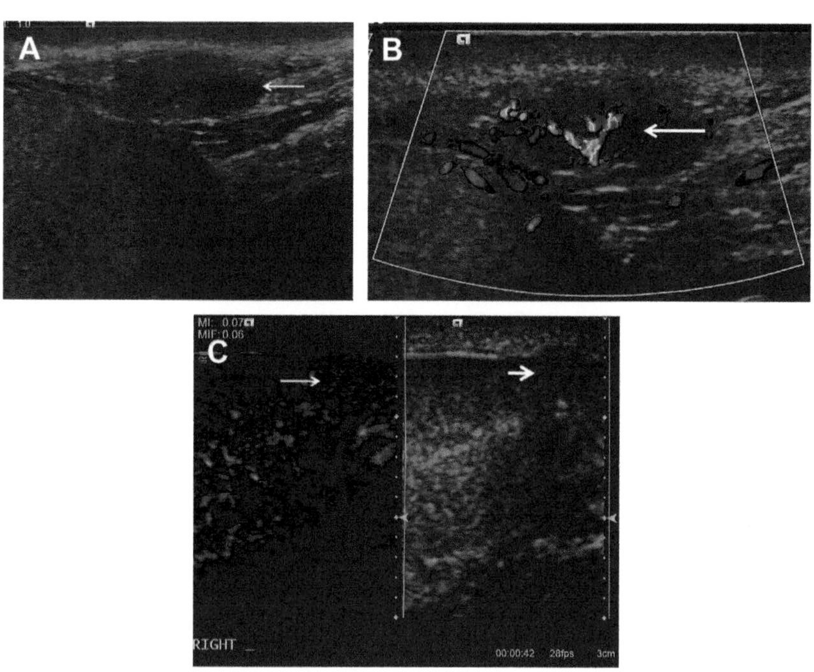

Fig. 13. Extratesticular adenomatoid lesion. (*A*) An isoreflective lesion is noted within the epididymis (*arrow*). (*B*) The lesion demonstrates increased color Doppler signal (*arrow*). (*C*) On contrast-enhanced ultrasonography, the epididymal lesion identified on B-Mode sonography (*short arrow*) demonstrates enhancement (*long arrow*) and early washout.

prompt surgical management.[48] However, exploration is not without risks, with testicular infection, atrophy, or necrosis all recognized complications.[71] CEUS allows exact preoperative evaluation by clearly defining viable tissue, and facilitates tissue-sparing surgery as opposed to complete orchidectomy.[15,55]

EXTRATESTICULAR LESIONS

Epididymal cysts are the most frequently encountered extratesticular lesion, with solid tumors being rare. Most primary extratesticular tumors in adults are benign: adenomatoid tumors are the most common, followed by lipomas (**Fig. 13**).[72,73] In children, rhabdomyosarcoma, although rare, must always be considered. The sonographic appearance of an adenomatoid tumor consists of a hyperechoic, rounded tumor, most commonly within the epididymal tail.[73] Following CEUS the focal epididymal lesion demonstrates enhancement and early washout of microbubble contrast.

SUMMARY

The use of high-frequency B-mode sonography and CDUS for the evaluation of scrotal abnormalities is well established. More recently, newer techniques such as CEUS have improved assessment by providing supplementary information in

cases where conventional techniques have been found wanting. By demonstrating the microcirculation in real time, CEUS allows a more clearly defined assessment of both acute and nonacute scrotal abnormalities. Increasing experience of this technique should therefore be advocated to enable greater operator confidence in diagnosis. This improvement may then facilitate more informed recommendations of close follow-up or targeted biopsy for conditions that currently undergo unnecessary orchidectomy.

REFERENCES

1. Rifkin MD, Kurtz AB, Pasto ME, et al. Diagnostic capabilities of high-resolution scrotal ultrasonography: prospective evaluation. J Ultrasound Med 1985;4:13–9.
2. Muller T, Gozzi C, Akkad T, et al. Management of incidental impalpable intratesticular masses of < or = 5 mm in diameter. BJU Int 2006;98:1001–4.
3. Schwerk WB, Schwerk WN, Rodeck G. Testicular tumors: prospective analysis of real-time US patterns and abdominal staging. Radiology 1987; 164:369–74.
4. Piscaglia F, Nolsoe C, Dietrich C, et al. The EF-SUMB guidelines and recommendations on the clinical practice of Contrast Enhanced Ultrasound (CEUS). Update 2011 on non-hepatic applications. Ultraschall Med 2012;1:11–2.

5. Piscaglia F, Bolondi L. The safety of Sonovue in abdominal applications: retrospective analysis of 23188 investigations. Ultrasound Med Biol 2006; 32:1369–75.
6. Dogra VS, Gottlieb RH, Oka M, et al. Sonography of the scrotum. Radiology 2003;227:18–36.
7. Middleton WD, Meredith MW. Analysis of intratesticular arterial anatomy with emphasis on transmediastinal arteries. Radiology 1993;189:157–60.
8. Harvey CJ, Blomley MJ, Eckersley RJ, et al. Developments in ultrasound contrast media. Eur Radiol 2001;11:675–89.
9. Cosgrove D. Developments in ultrasound. Imaging 2006;18:82–96.
10. Harvey CJ, Sidhu PS. Ultrasound contrast agents in genito-urinary imaging. Ultrasound Clin North Am 2011;5:489–506.
11. Simpson DH, Chin CT, Burns PN. Pulse inversion Doppler: a new method for detecting nonlinear echoes from microbubble contrast agents. IEEE Trans Biomed Eng 1999;46:372–82.
12. Eckersley RJ, Chin CT, Burns PN. Optimising phase and amplitude modulation schemes for imaging microbubble contrast agents at low acoustic power. Ultrasound Med Biol 2005;31:213–9.
13. Wilson SR, Burns PN. Microbubble-enhanced US in body imaging: what role? Radiology 2010;257:24–39.
14. Valentino M, Bertolotto M, Derchi L, et al. Role of contrast enhanced ultrasound in acute scrotal diseases. Eur Radiol 2011;21:1831–40.
15. Hedayati V, Sellars ME, Sharma DM, et al. Contrast-enhanced ultrasound in testicular trauma: role in directing exploration, debridement and organ salvage. Br J Radiol 2012;85:e65–8.
16. Lung PF, Jaffer OS, Sellars ME, et al. Contrast enhanced ultrasound (CEUS) in the evaluation of focal testicular complications secondary to epididymitis. AJR Am J Roentgenol 2012;199:W345–54.
17. Dietrich CF, Ignee A, Hocke M, et al. Pitfalls and artefacts using contrast enhanced ultrasound. Z Gastroenterol 2011;49:350–6.
18. Greenlee RT, Hill-Harmon MB, Murray T, et al. Cancer statistics, 2001. CA Cancer J Clin 2001;1(51):15–36.
19. Sidhu PS. The EFSUMB guidelines for contrast-enhanced ultrasound are comprehensive and informative for good clinical practice: will radiologists take the lead? Br J Radiol 2008;81:524–5.
20. Patel K, Sellars ME, Clarke JL, et al. Features of testicular epidermoid cysts on contrast enhanced ultrasound and real time elastography. J Ultrasound Med 2012;31:1115–22.
21. Lock G, Schmidt C, Helmich F, et al. Early experience with contrast enhanced ultrasound in the diagnosis of testicular masses; a feasibility study. Urology 2011;77:1049–53.
22. Horstman WG, Melson GL, Middleton WD, et al. Testicular tumors: findings with color Doppler US. Radiology 1992;185:733–7.
23. Mostofi FK, Sesterhenn IA, Davis CJ. Immunopathology of germ cell tumors of the testis. Semin Diagn Pathol 1987;4:320–41.
24. Verhoeven RH, Gondos A, Janssen-Heijnen ML, et al. Testicular cancer in Europe and the USA: survival still rising among older patients. Ann Oncol 2013;24:508–13.
25. Woodward PJ, Sohaey R, O'Donoghue MJ, et al. Tumors and tumorlike lesions of the testis: radiologic-pathologic correlation. Radiographics 2002;22:189–216.
26. Lung PF, Sidhu PS. Scrotal masses: benign and malignant. Ultrasound Clin North Am 2011;5:443–56.
27. Huang DY, Sidhu PS. Focal testicular lesions: colour Doppler ultrasound, contrast-enhanced ultrasound and tissue elastography as adjuvants to the diagnosis. Br J Radiol 2012;85:S41–53.
28. Geraghty MJ, Lee FT Jr, Bernsten SA, et al. Sonography of testicular tumors and tumor-like conditions: a radiologic-pathologic correlation. Crit Rev Diagn Imaging 1998;39:1–63.
29. Bahrami A, Ro JY, Ayala AG. An overview of testicular germ cell tumors. Arch Pathol Lab Med 2007;131:1267–80.
30. Lee SC, Kim KH, Kim SH, et al. Mixed testicular germ cell tumor presenting as metastatic pure choriocarcinoma involving multiple lung metastases that was effectively treated with high-dose chemotherapy. Cancer Res Treat 2009;41:229–32.
31. Cao D, Humphrey PA. Yolk sac tumor of the testis. J Urol 2011;186:1475–6.
32. Luker GD, Siegel MJ. Pediatric testicular tumors: evaluation with gray-scale and color Doppler US. Radiology 1994;191:561–4.
33. Frush DP, Sheldon CA. Diagnostic imaging for pediatric scrotal disorders. Radiographics 1998;18:969–85.
34. Xu HX, Yi XP. Sonographic appearance of a testicular yolk sac tumor in a 2-year-old boy. J Clin Ultrasound 2007;35:55–7.
35. Kim I, Young RH, Scully RE. Leydig cell tumors of the testis: a clinicopathological analysis of 40 cases and review of the literature. Am J Surg Pathol 1985;9:177–92.
36. Avery GR, Peakman DJ, Young JR. Unusual hyperechoic ultrasound appearance of testicular Leydig cell tumor. Clin Radiol 1991;43:260–1.
37. Maizlin ZV, Belenky A, Kunichezky M, et al. Leydig cell tumors of the testis: gray scale and color doppler sonographic appearance. J Ultrasound Med 2004;23:959–64.
38. Lui P, Thorner P. Sonographic appearance of Sertoli cell tumor with pathologic correlation. Pediatr Radiol 1993;23:127–8.

39. Doll DC, Weiss RB. Malignant lymphoma of the testis. Am J Med 1986;81:515–23.
40. Horne MJ, Adeniran AJ. Primary diffuse large B-cell lymphoma of the testis. Arch Pathol Lab Med 2011;135:1363–7.
41. Tweed CS, Peck RJ. A sonographic appearance of testicular lymphoma. Clin Radiol 1991;43:341–2.
42. Ferry JA, Harris NL, Young RH, et al. Malignant lymphoma of the testis, epididymis, and spermatic cord. A clinicopathologic study of 69 cases with immunophenotypic analysis. Am J Surg Pathol 1994;18:376–90.
43. Mazzu D, Jeffrey RB, Ralls PW. Lymphoma and leukaemia involving the testicles: findings on gray-scale and color Doppler sonography. AJR Am J Roentgenol 1995;164:645–7.
44. Emura A, Kudo S, Mihara M, et al. Testicular malignant lymphoma; imaging and diagnosis. Radiat Med 1996;14:121–6.
45. Rayor RA, Scheible W, Brock WA, et al. High resolution ultrasonography in the diagnosis of testicular relapse in patients with acute lymphoblastic leukaemia. J Urol 1982;128:602–3.
46. Garcia-Gonzalez R, Pinto J, Val-Bernal JF. Testicular metastases from solid tumors: an autopsy study. Ann Diagn Pathol 2000;4:397–400.
47. Atchley JT, Dewbury KC. Ultrasound appearances of testicular epidermoid cysts. Clin Radiol 2000;55:493–502.
48. Stewart VR, Sidhu PS. The testis: the unusual, the rare and the bizarre. Clin Radiol 2007;62:289–302.
49. Langer JE, Ramchandani P, Siegelman ES, et al. Epidermoid cysts of the testicle: sonographic and MR imaging features. Am J Roentgenol 1999;173:1295–9.
50. Sidhu PS, Allan PL, Cattin F, et al. Diagnostic efficacy of Sonovue(R), a second generation contrast agent, in the assessment of extracranial carotid or peripheral arteries using colour and spectral Doppler ultrasound: a multicentre study. Br J Radiol 2006;79:44–51.
51. Rouviere O, Bouvier R, Pangaud C, et al. Tubular ectasia of the rete testis: a potential pitfall in scrotal imaging. Eur Radiol 1999;9:1862–8.
52. Mellick LB. Torsion of the testicle: it is time to stop tossing the dice. Pediatr Emerg Care 2012;28:80–6.
53. Dubinsky TJ, Chen P, Maklad N. Color-flow and power doppler imaging of the testes. World J Urol 1998;16:35–40.
54. Cokkinos DD, Antypa E, Kalogeropoulos I, et al. Contrast-enhanced ultrasound performed under urgent conditions. Indications, review of the technique, clinical examples and limitations. Insights Imaging 2013;4:185–98.
55. Moschouris H, Stamatiou K, Lampropoulou E, et al. Imaging of the acute scrotum; is there a place for contrast-enhanced ultrasonography. Int Braz J Urol 2009;35:702–5.
56. Sidhu PS. Clinical and imaging features of testicular torsion: role of ultrasound. Clin Radiol 1999;54:343–52.
57. Corriere JN. Horizontal lie of the testicle: a diagnostic sign and torsion of the testis. J Urol 1972;107:616–7.
58. Bird K, Rosenfield AT, Taylor KJ. Ultrasonography in testicular torsion. Radiology 1983;147:527–34.
59. Vijayaraghavan SB. Sonographic differential diagnosis of acute scrotum: real-time whirlpool sign, a key sign of torsion. J Ultrasound Med 2006;25:563–74.
60. Lerner RG, Mevorach RA, Hulbert WC, et al. Color Doppler US in the evaluation of acute scrotal disease. Radiology 1990;176:355–8.
61. Albrecht T, Lotzof K, Hussain HK, et al. Power Doppler US of the normal prepubertal testis: does it live up to its promises? Radiology 1997;203:227–31.
62. Bilagi P, Sriprasad S, Clarke J, et al. Clinical and ultrasound features of segmental testicular infarction: six-year experience from a single centre. Eur Radiol 2007;17:2810–8.
63. Fernandez-Perez GC, Tardaguila FM, Velasco M, et al. Radiologic findings of segmental testicular infarction. Am J Roentgenol 2005;184:1587–93.
64. Bertolotto M, Derchi LE, Sidhu PS, et al. Acute segmental testicular infarction at contrast-enhanced ultrasound: early features and changes during follow-up. AJR Am J Roentgenol 2011;196:834–41.
65. Wu VH, Dangman BC, Kayfman RP. Sonographic appearance of acute testicular venous infarction in a patient with hypercoagulable state. J Ultrasound Med 1995;14:57–9.
66. Bird K, Rosenfield AT. Testicular infarction secondary to acute inflammatory disease: demonstration by B-scan ultrasound. Radiology 1984;152:785–8.
67. Dogra VS, Gottlieb RH, Rubens DJ, et al. Benign intratesticular cystic lesions: US features. Radiographics 2001;21:S273–81.
68. Sidhu PS, Sriprasad S, Bushby LH, et al. Impalpable testis cancer. BJU Int 2004;93:888.
69. Dogra VS, Bhatt S. Acute painful scrotum. Radiol Clin North Am 2004;42:349–63.
70. Horstman WG, Middleton WD, Melson GL. Scrotal inflammatory disease: color Doppler US findings. Radiology 1991;179:55–9.
71. Buckley JC, McAninch JW. Use of ultrasound for the diagnosis of testicular injuries in blunt scrotal trauma. J Urol 2006;175:175–8.
72. Woodward PJ, Schwab CM, Sesterhenn IA. Extratesticular scrotal masses: radiologic-pathologic correlation. Radiographics 2003;23:215–40.
73. Akbar SA, Sayyed TA, Jafri SZ, et al. Multimodality imaging of paratesticular neoplasms and their rare mimics. Radiographics 2003;23:1461–76.

Testicular Trauma
Role of Sonography

Refky Nicola, MS, DO, Nancy Carson, MBA, RDMS, RVT, Vikram Dogra, MD*

KEYWORDS

• Scrotal trauma • Testis • Ultrasonography

KEY POINTS

- High-frequency ultrasonography is the modality of choice for the evaluation of scrotal trauma.
- It is cost-effective, uses nonionizing radiation, is readily available, and portable.
- Color flow Doppler imaging is invaluable in that it allows for the assessment of any associated vascular injury.
- Ultrasonographic examination can help diagnose testicular rupture, testicular torsion, hematoceles, and hematomas.
- In more than 80% of cases, ruptured testes are salvageable with surgical intervention in the first 72 hours.

INTRODUCTION

The management of scrotal trauma requires a careful physical examination and a reliable imaging modality to maximize positive outcomes. A physical examination can be difficult in the setting of trauma, secondary to severe pain and scrotal swelling. Therefore, high-frequency ultrasonography (US) has become a reliable modality in the evaluation of intratesticular and extratesticular injuries. This modality allows for appropriate triaging of patients for medical and possibly immediate surgical management.

There are several benefits to the use of US, ranging from low cost compared with other cross-sectional modalities to its ease of availability. Positive US findings may indicate the need for urgent surgical intervention; however, negative US findings should not prevent surgical exploration if there is a high degree of suspicion for testicular fracture.[1]

Sonographic Scrotal and Testicular Anatomy

The scrotum comprises several layers consisting of the following from superficial to deep: the rugated skin, superficial fascia, dartos muscle, external spermatic fascia, cremasteric fascia and muscle, and internal spermatic fascia. The normal thickness of the scrotal wall ranges from approximately 2 to 8 mm, depending on the level of contraction of the cremasteric muscle.[2]

The testes are separated from the scrotum by the visceral and parietal layers of the tunica vaginalis. These 2 layers join at a small area on the posterior testis, where they also attach to the scrotal wall. A few millimeters of fluid are normally found in the potential space between the visceral and parietal tunica vaginalis. The average adult testes measures approximately 5 × 3 × 2 cm. The parenchyma consists of multiple lobules, containing many seminiferous tubule that lead to dilated spaces of the rete testes in the mediastinum. The mediastinum of the testes appears as a horizontal echogenic band on longitudinal grayscale images, and should not be mistaken for a pathologic lesion (**Fig. 1**).

The epididymis consists of the head, body, and tail. The head arises from the superior aspect of the testes; the body and tail extend inferolaterally. The tail continues on as the vas deferens as it

Department of Imaging Sciences, University of Rochester Medical Center, 601 Elmwood Avenue, PO Box 648, Rochester, NY 14642, USA
* Corresponding author.
E-mail address: vikram_dogra@umrc.rochester.edu

Ultrasound Clin 8 (2013) 525–530
http://dx.doi.org/10.1016/j.cult.2013.07.004
1556-858X/13/$ – see front matter © 2013 Elsevier Inc. All rights reserved.

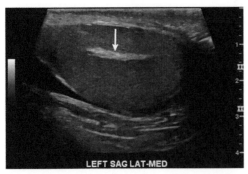

Fig. 1. Mediastinum testis. Longitudinal grayscale image of a normal testis demonstrates a linear echogenic band (*arrow*) along the long axis of the testis, known as the mediastinum testis.

merges with the spermatic cord. The epididymal head measures approximately 10 to 12 mm and the body is less than 4 mm in thickness. The epididymis should be isoechoic to hypoechoic compared with the testicular parenchyma.

Sonographic Technique of the Scrotum

Evaluation of the scrotum is best done with the patient in the supine position, with the scrotum elevated and supported with a towel between the thighs. Post-traumatic pain and swelling can make the examination difficult. A 7 to 14 MHz high-frequency linear array transducer is ideal for fine detail; however, scrotal enlargement from various causes may require using a curved, lower-frequency transducer for better penetration. If possible, the evaluation of the asymptomatic side is recommended first, using that side to set the technical parameters for the grayscale and color flow Doppler evaluation of both testes. Transverse side-by-side images showing both testes are essential for finding subtle differences in blood flow and echogenicity (**Fig. 2**). The presence of intratesticular arterial and venous blood flow is documented in each testis using spectral and color Doppler. Each testis should have 3 spectral

Doppler images recorded: upper, mid, and lower pole. Spectral Doppler waveforms in the testicular artery and epididymis normally have a characteristic low-resistance pattern (**Fig. 3**).[3]

Mechanism of Scrotal Injury

Several factors help protect the testes from blunt trauma. The testes are highly mobile in the lax skin of the scrotum, allowing them to slide away from impact. The testes are also protected by the tunica albuginea, which forms a tough capsule around the organ. The common mechanism of injury is when the testes is caught and crushed between the thigh and perineum or against the symphysis pubis. The most common cause of blunt trauma is sports-related injury, accounting for more than half of all blunt scrotal trauma; the second most common cause is motor vehicle collision, accounting for 9% to 17%.[4] Penetrating scrotal trauma is rare and is mainly associated with gunshot wounds; other causes include bite or stab wounds. Bilateral blunt injury is rare, only seen in 1.5% of cases, but is found to be higher in the setting of penetrating injury at about 30% of cases.[5,6]

Iatrogenic injury can sometimes occur from scrotal surgery, hernia repair, or orchiectomy. The main complications are infection and nerve injury, but severe injury such as transection of the spermatic cord can occur rarely, leading to large hematoceles and progressing scrotal edema.[7,8]

EXTRATESTICULAR FINDINGS OF SCROTAL TRAUMA
Hematocele

Hematocele is blood in the space between the layers of the tunica vaginalis, and is the most common finding in testicular trauma. It can be an indicator of intratesticular or extratesticular injury, but can also be present as an isolated finding. As a hematocele ages, its appearance changes. An

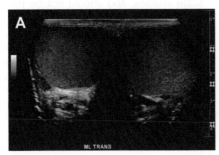

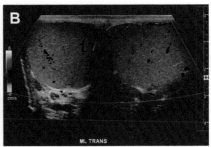

Fig. 2. Normal testis. (*A*) Grayscale and (*B*) color flow Doppler transverse images of both testes demonstrate homogeneous echotexture and symmetric blood flow.

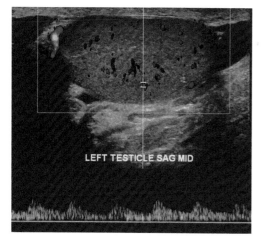

Fig. 3. Normal arterial flow. Sagittal color and spectral Doppler image demonstrates a normal low-resistance arterial waveform from a left testicle.

acute hematocele appears echogenic and over time may develop any or all of the following: fluid-fluid levels, debris, and reticular septations (**Fig. 4**).[9] A large hematocele can potentially mask other important findings in the scrotum, making disruption of the tunica albuginea difficult to exclude. For these reasons, the presence of a large hematocele necessitates surgical exploration, despite the lack of US evidence of tunica albuginea rupture.

Hematoma of the Scrotal Wall

Scrotal wall hematoma appears as thickening of the scrotal wall, with decreased or absent Doppler

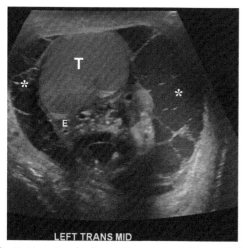

Fig. 4. Hematocele. Grayscale transverse image of the left testis taken as a follow-up at 7 days after scrotal trauma demonstrates a hematocele (*asterisk*) with septations. E, epididymis; T, testis.

flow (**Fig. 5**). It is a common finding in blunt testicular injury, and is often associated with hematocele or intratesticular hematoma. Typically, scrotal wall hematomas resolve spontaneously or with conservative management.

Traumatic Epididymitis

Traumatic epididymitis has a similar appearance to infectious epididymitis. The epididymis is enlarged, has heterogeneous echotexture, and has increased vascularity on color Doppler. The heterogeneous echotexture is caused by hematomas and contusion, which may be localized or include the entire epididymis. These findings can mimic epididymitis caused by *Escherichia coli* or *Proteus* sp., but the history of trauma differentiates the 2 causes.[10]

Epididymal Fracture

Although less common than traumatic epididymitis, epididymal fracture may be seen with testicular traumatic injuries. Much like testicular fracture, epididymal fractures appear as areas of avascularity with heterogeneous echotexture in an overall ill-defined epididymis. This type of injury is rarely seen on the US examination. It is usually diagnosed during surgical exploration for testicular rupture or large hematomas, as concurrent hematoceles can obscure subtle injury to the epididymis.

Hematoma of the Spermatic Cord

Hematomas of the spermatic cord most commonly arise in patients who have undergone surgery for inguinal hernia. A hematoma in the spermatic cord is usually caused by injury to the spermatic cord vessels, such as rupture of a varicocele due to blunt trauma. These hematomas lie within the

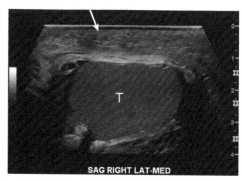

Fig. 5. Hematoma of the scrotal wall. Ultrasonographic grayscale image of a patient presenting after a sports injury demonstrates diffuse scrotal wall thickening (*arrow*) secondary to hemorrhage. There is no injury to the testis (T).

tunica vaginalis. On US examination, a hematoma of the spermatic cord appears as a well-defined heterogeneous avascular mass superior to the testis. It is possible to have spermatic cord hematomas that do not arise from the scrotum, but they are really extensions of retroperitoneal hematomas.[11]

INTRATESTICULAR FINDINGS OF SCROTAL TRAUMA
Traumatic Testicular Torsion

It has been reported that 4% to 8% of testicular torsions are secondary to acute trauma.[12] Traumatic testicular torsion has a similar US appearance to the more common nontraumatic torsion of the spermatic cord. Prompt diagnosis and surgical intervention allow maximal salvage rates of the torsed testicle. Color Doppler imaging of the torsed testicle demonstrates absent flow in the affected testes, and a swirling appearance of the vessels of the spermatic cord can sometimes be seen. Homogeneous parenchyma, without signs of necrosis or infarction, indicates that the testis can be salvaged.[13]

Testicular Fracture

Testicular fracture refers to discontinuity of the normal testicular parenchyma. On US examination, the fracture line appears as a hypoechoic avascular area. The presence of vascularity by color Doppler indicates viable tissue.[14] Testicular fracture lines may occur with or without an intact tunica albuginea and treatment may be conservative, depending on the size of the avascular area.

Testicular Rupture

US plays a significant role in the early diagnosis of testicular rupture, allowing maximization of salvage rates secondary to prompt surgical repair. Sensitivity of 100% and specificity of 65% to 93.5% have been obtained in US detection of rupture in separate series.[15,16]

On US examination, the tunica albuginea normally appears as 2 parallel hyperechoic lines surrounding the testis. An intact tunica albuginea confidently excludes testicular rupture; in the clinical setting of trauma, discontinuity of the tunica albuginea on US examination indicates testicular rupture. Other US findings that increase confidence in a diagnosis of testicular rupture in order of importance are contour abnormality, heterogeneous parenchymal echotexture, and avascular areas in the testes. These findings in combination with discontinuity of the tunica albuginea are highly sensitive and specific for testicular rupture.[14–16]

Contour abnormality in the ruptured testis is caused by extrusion of parenchyma from the defect in the tunica albuginea.[13] This can be seen on US examination as a kink or bulge in the normally smooth curvilinear tunica albuginea covering the testes (**Fig. 6**). When a large hematocele or scrotal swelling from a large wall hematoma limits evaluation of the integrity of the tunica albuginea, a contour abnormality is considered indirect evidence of rupture.

In more than 80% of cases, ruptured testes can be salvaged by surgical repair within the first 72 hours after injury.[16] Surgical exploration cannot be avoided if there is a large hematocele, which can obscure the tunica albuginea, and limit confidence in its integrity.[17,18]

Intratesticular Hematoma

Intratesticular hematomas are a common finding in scrotal trauma, and are found to be of variable size and number. Acute hematomas can have variable appearance on initial examination, ranging from

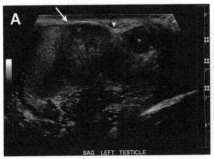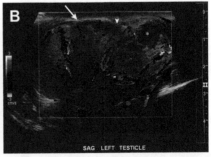

Fig. 6. Testicular rupture. (*A*) Grayscale and (*B*) color flow Doppler images of a 42-year-old patient who was in a motor vehicle collision demonstrate disruption (*arrowhead*) of tunica albuginea (*arrow*). There is loss of vascularity within the ruptured segment of the testis, a contour abnormality of the testis, and extrusion of testicular tissue (*asterisk*) within the left scrotum. The patient was taken immediately for surgical exploration and underwent an orchiectomy.

nearly isoechoic to the normal testicular parenchyma, to a subtle diffuse heterogeneity (**Fig. 7**). Like hematomas elsewhere, intratesticular hematomas shrink in size with time and become hypoechoic to anechoic. The primary role of the US examination is to evaluate for testicular ruptures that need surgical management from small hematomas with an intact tunica; which can be treated with nonsteroidal anti-inflammatory drugs, icepacks, and serial follow-up examinations. A hematoma does not demonstrate vascularity on the US examination. Up to 10% to 15% of testicular neoplasms are first found incidentally on US examination for other indications,[14] therefore any intrastesticular lesion found in a patient with trauma needs to be followed by US to demonstrate its complete resolution to exclude underlying malignancy.

It is important to re-evaluate acute intratesticular hematomas in the first 12 to 24 hours after the initial examination to diagnose hematomas that may have been missed on the initial examination secondary to a subtle appearance or isoechogenicity to normal parenchyma. Continued follow-up of conservatively treated hematomas is required because up to 40% develop infection and necrosis, possibly needing an orchiectomy.[14] As infection develops, the hematoma remains avascular on Doppler US, but develops surrounding peripheral hyperemia.[19]

Intratesticular Pseudoaneurysm

Intratesticular pseudoaneurysm is a rare complication of either blunt or penetrating trauma.[20] The intratesticular pseudoaneurysm appears similar to pseudoaneurysms elsewhere in the body, characterized by anechoic areas with active vascularity on color and spectral Doppler. These pseudoaneurysms have the yin-yang or to-and fro sign on spectral Doppler examination. Differential diagnosis includes an incidental intratesticular varicocele, which shows a venous waveform on spectral Doppler that increases with Valsalva, versus the to-and-fro (yin-yang sign) flow pattern of the pseudoaneurysm.[20,21] Treatment of intratesticular pseudoaneurysms can vary from surgery or angiographic embolization to conservative management.[20]

Testicular Dislocation

Posttraumatic testicular dislocation can occur to any nearby space. The inguinal canal is the most common site, occurring in 50% of cases; the other possible sites of testicular dislocation include pubic (18%), canalicular (8%), penile (8%), intraabdominal (6%), perineal (4%), and crural (2%).[22] A common history involves direct impact to the groin from motorcycle fuel tanks.[23] Early detection of testicular dislocation is important to decrease the chance of permanent changes to the testes, such as atrophy, impaired spermatogenesis, or malignant degeneration.[24,25]

Penetrating Trauma

As in blunt trauma, US is valuable in determining the severity of penetrating trauma so that proper management can be implemented. Nearly all penetrating injuries to the scrotum are from gunshot wounds. Physical examination can clearly show entrance wounds, with or without exit wounds. On the US examination, intrascrotal locules of air are commonly seen and appear as multiple echogenic foci with dirty shadowing from the reverberation artifact. If present in the testes or scrotal tissues, missile fragments appear as bright echogenic foci. Plain radiography and computed tomography can help detect and/or differentiate metallic foreign bodies from intrascrotal air if the results of US are unclear. Hematocele and scrotal wall hematoma may be seen, with or without actual disruption of the testes. Bullet tracks in the testicular parenchyma will appear as hypoechogenic linear areas with decreased flow. Color

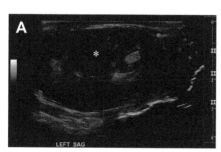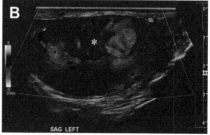

Fig. 7. Testicular hematoma. (*A*) Longitudinal grayscale and (*B*) color flow Doppler images of a 22-year-old patient with scrotal trauma as result of a motor vehicle collision demonstrate a hypoechoic avascular region within the testis (*asterisk*) suggestive of intratesticular hematoma. The absence of color flow Doppler favors an intratesticular hematoma.

Doppler imaging helps determine viable tissue from avascular tissue needing surgical debridement and closure.[25] Management is similar to that of blunt trauma. A large hematocele may obscure associated testicular or epididymal injury, and warrant surgical exploration.

Animal or human bites are a rare cause of penetrating trauma, and are of greater concern for development of posttraumatic infection.[26–28]

SUMMARY

High-frequency US is the modality of choice for the evaluation of scrotal trauma. It is cost-effective, uses nonionizing radiation, is readily available, and portable. Color flow Doppler imaging is invaluable in that it allows for the assessment of any associated vascular injury. US examination can help diagnose testicular rupture, testicular torsion, hematoceles, and hematomas, thus helping triage patients for immediate surgical intervention or medical management. In more than 80% of cases, ruptured testes are salvageable with surgical intervention in the first 72 hours.

REFERENCES

1. Mulhall JP, Gabram SG, Jacobs LM. Emergency management of blunt testicular trauma. Acad Emerg Med 1995;2(7):639–43.
2. Hricak H, Filly RA. Sonography of the scrotum. Invest Radiol 1983;18(2):112–21.
3. Oyen RH. Scrotal ultrasound. Eur Radiol 2002;12(1):19–34.
4. Haas CA, Brown SL, Spirnak JP. Penile fracture and testicular rupture. World J Urol 1999;17(2):101–6.
5. Cass AS, Ferrara L, Wolpert J, et al. Bilateral testicular injury from external trauma. J Urol 1988;140(6):1435–6.
6. Cass AS, Luxenberg M. Testicular injuries. Urology 1991;37(6):528–30.
7. Ridgway PF, Shah J, Darzi AW. Male genital tract injuries after contemporary inguinal hernia repair. BJU Int 2002;90(3):272–6.
8. Taylor EW, Duffy K, Lee K, et al. Surgical site infection after groin hernia repair. Br J Surg 2004;91(1):105–11.
9. Haddad FS, Manne RK, Nathan MH. The pathological, ultrasonographic and computerized tomographic characteristics of chronic hematocele. J Urol 1988;139(3):594–5.
10. Gordon LM, Stein SM, Ralls PW. Traumatic epididymitis: evaluation with color Doppler sonography. AJR Am J Roentgenol 1996;166:1323–5.
11. McKenney MG, Fietsam R Jr, Glover JL, et al. Spermatic cord hematoma: case report and literature review. Am Surg 1996;62(9):768–9.
12. Seng YJ, Moissinac K. Trauma induced testicular torsion: a reminder for the unwary. J Accid Emerg Med 2000;17(5):381–2.
13. Dogra V, Bhatt S. Acute painful scrotum. Radiol Clin North Am 2004;42(2):349–63.
14. Deurdulian C, Mittelstaedt CA, Chong WK, et al. US of acute scrotal trauma: optimal technique, imaging findings, and management. Radiographics 2007;27(2):357–69.
15. Guichard G, El Ammari J, Del Coro C, et al. Accuracy of ultrasonography in diagnosis of testicular rupture after blunt scrotal trauma. Urology 2008;71(1):52–6.
16. Buckley JC, McAninch JW. Use of ultrasonography for the diagnosis of testicular injuries in blunt scrotal trauma. J Urol 2006;175(1):175–8.
17. Altarac S. Management of 53 cases of testicular trauma. Eur Urol 1994;25(2):119–23.
18. Corrales JG, Corbel L, Cipolla B, et al. Accuracy of ultrasound diagnosis after blunt testicular trauma. J Urol 1993;150(6):1834–6.
19. Dogra VS, Gottlieb RH, Oka M, et al. Sonography of the scrotum. Radiology 2003;227(1):18–36.
20. Dee KE, Deck AJ, Waitches GM. Intratesticular pseudoaneurysm after blunt trauma. AJR Am J Roentgenol 2000;174(4):1136.
21. Mehta AL, Dogra VS. Intratesticular varicocele. J Clin Ultrasound 1998;26(1):49–51.
22. Schwartz SL, Faerber GJ. Dislocation of the testis as a delayed presentation of scrotal trauma. Urology 1994;43(5):743–5.
23. Ihama Y, Fuke C, Miyazaki T. A two-rider motorcycle accident involving injuries around groin area in both the driver and the passenger. Leg Med 2007;9(5):274–7.
24. Bromberg W, Wong C, Kurek S, et al. Traumatic bilateral testicular dislocation. J Trauma 2003;54(5):1009–11.
25. Learch TJ, Hansch LP, Ralls PW. Sonography in patients with gunshot wounds of the scrotum: imaging findings and their value. AJR Am J Roentgenol 1995;165(4):879–83.
26. Dubosq F, Traxer O, Boublil V, et al. Management of dog bite trauma of the external genital organs. Prog Urol 2004;14(2):232–3.
27. Cummings P. Antibiotics to prevent infection in patients with dog bite wounds: a meta-analysis of randomized trials. Ann Emerg Med 1994;23(3):535–40.
28. Kerins M, Greene S, O'Connor N. A human bite to the scrotum: a case report and review of the literature. Eur J Emerg Med 2004;11(4):223–4.

The Acute Scrotum

Lorenzo E. Derchi, MD[a],*, Michele Bertolotto, MD[b],
Massimo Valentino, MD[c], Alchiede Simonato, MD[d]

KEYWORDS

- Acute scrotum • Imaging • Testicular torsion • Orchitis • Epididymitis

KEY POINTS

- Clinical history and physical examination do not always allow a firm differential among the different possible cause of acute scrotum, and imaging is needed to provide a diagnosis.
- Differentiating torsion from infection is a clinical emergency.
- Inflammatory conditions of the scrotum are the most frequent cause of acute scrotal pain in the adult population.
- The acute scrotum has several less common causes.

An acute scrotum, defined as acute painful swelling of the scrotum, is a common cause of presentation to the emergency department. A large variety of pathologic conditions must be considered: torsion, infection, trauma, incarcerated inguinal hernia, segmental infarction, hemorrhage, vasculitis, and complications after hernia surgery.[1-3] Torsion and infection are by far the most common causes of acute scrotum; infection is more frequent in adults, whereas torsion (either of the testis or of a testicular appendage) is more common in children.[3]

Clinical history and physical examination do not always allow a firm differential among the different possible cause of acute scrotum, and imaging is needed to provide a diagnosis. High-resolution ultrasonography is the preferred modality for evaluating the acute scrotum.[4] It allows delineation of the anatomic details of the testis and, with the help of Doppler techniques, provides information about scrotal perfusion changes. It is then possible, in most cases, to reach a correct diagnosis and guide proper treatment. In selected patients, especially to provide unequivocal differentiation between hypovascular and avascular focal testicular lesions, contrast-enhanced ultrasonography has proven useful.[5]

This article outlines the ultrasonographic and Doppler findings in patients with acute scrotum of nontraumatic origin.

TESTICULAR TORSION

Differentiating torsion from infection is a clinical emergency. Depending on the degree of torsion, testicular infarction may in fact develop within a short time, and rapid intervention is needed. Clinical history and scrotal examination may not reveal the classical signs of torsion, and imaging is necessary to provide a differential between torsion and infection or other causes of acute scrotum. Testicular salvage rate depends on 2 factors: the duration of ischemia and the degree of torsion. Detorsion has an almost 100% salvage rate if it occurs within 6 hours from the onset of symptoms, a 70% rate if occurring between 6 and 12 hours, and a 20% rate if occurring within 12 to 24 hours. The degree of torsion may vary from 180° to 720° or more. A low-grade torsed spermatic cord may cause testicular infarction in a relatively long time through a mechanism starting with venous and lymphatic obstruction, followed by arterial occlusion; high-grade torsions directly induce arterial occlusion and lead to testicular infarction in a few hours.[1-3]

[a] Department of Radiology, University of Genoa, IRCCS Azienda Ospedaliera Universitaria San Martino IST, Largo R. Benzi 10, I-16132, Genoa, Italy; [b] Department of Radiology, University of Trieste, Ospedale di Cattinara, Strada di Fiume 447, I-3449, Trieste, Italy; [c] Department of Radiology, Ospedale di Tolmezzo, Via Morgagni 18, I-33028, Tolmezzo (Udine), Italy; [d] Department of Urology, University of Genoa, IRCCS Azienda Ospedaliera Universitaria San Martino IST, Largo R. Benzi 10, I-16132, Genoa, Italy
* Corresponding author.
E-mail address: 54464@unige.it

Ultrasound Clin 8 (2013) 531–544
http://dx.doi.org/10.1016/j.cult.2013.06.001
1556-858X/13/$ – see front matter © 2013 Elsevier Inc. All rights reserved.

The 2 types of torsion are extravaginal and intravaginal.

Extravaginal Torsion

Extravaginal torsion of the spermatic cord occurs outside the tunica vaginalis, where the testis and gubernaculum are not fixed and are free to rotate. This condition occurs almost exclusively in utero or in newborns. The babies present with scrotal swelling, reddening of the skin, and a firm mass on the affected side, which must be considered a surgical emergency. A salvage rate up to 40% has been reported in some series in which prompt surgical treatment was performed.[6,7] At ultrasonography, the testis is enlarged and heterogeneous, with a thin peripheral hyperechogenic rim and lack of internal flow at Doppler study.[8] The Doppler examination needs proper technique (increasing the gain, decreasing the wall filter, decreasing the pulse repetition frequency, and using a high-frequency transducer), because parameters must be optimized to detect the slow flow signals within the neonatal testis. The contralateral testis can be used as a comparison (usually with axial scans in which portions of each testis are seen on the same image), but it must be remembered that torsion can be bilateral in up to 2% of cases.

Intravaginal Torsion

Intravaginal torsion of the spermatic cord occurs within the tunica vaginalis and is the most common type of torsion. It is more frequent in the adolescent age range but may be encountered in any age group. An increased risk of torsion is observed in patients with the so-called bell-clapper anomaly. In these cases, the tunica vaginalis testis is not attached to the posterolateral aspect of the testis, but completely encircles the testis, epididymis, and distal spermatic cord, thus predisposing the testis to torsion around the high point of attachment. The anomaly has a 12% prevalence

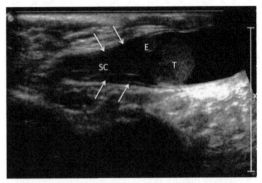

Fig. 1. Sagittal ultrasound of the left hemiscrotum in a 5-year-old boy with a hydrocele and the bell-clapper anomaly. A small amount of fluid (*arrows*) encircles the distal part of the spermatic cord. E, epididymis; SC, spermatic cord; T, testis.

and is bilateral in 89% of affected patients. It can be recognized through ultrasonography when a small amount of fluid encircles the distal part of the spermatic cord (**Fig. 1**).[1,2]

During the examination for suspected testicular torsion, the symptomatic testis should be compared with the contralateral one, because an asymmetry of findings is helpful to establish the diagnosis. However, care should always be taken, because intravaginal torsion also may be bilateral.

The gray-scale ultrasonographic findings at the testis are related to the period between onset of symptoms and the examination. Immediately after onset of pain, the involved testis may appear normal, but progressive development of edematous changes makes it hypoechogenic. At 4 to 6 hours, the testis is usually swollen and hypoechoic, whereas a heterogeneous structure develops at 24 hours, related to vascular congestion, hemorrhage, and necrosis (**Fig. 2A**).

Twisting of the spermatic cord at the external inguinal ring may be recognized. This twisting has been described as the "Whirlpool sign" and, when visible, is a highly specific sign of torsion.[9]

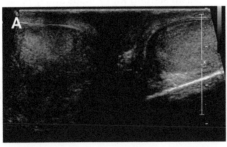
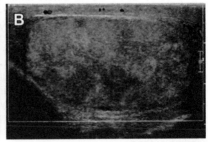

Fig. 2. (A) Ultrasound of the scrotum in a 27-year-old man who presented with acute pain in the right testis lasting 24 hours. (A) On axial image, the right testis is swollen, with a heterogeneous echotexture. (B) Intratesticular flow signals are absent and only a few vessels are visible within the scrotal wall. Torsion was confirmed at surgery.

Because gray-scale images are often normal in the first phases of torsion, Doppler techniques are needed to evaluate testicular perfusion changes. Although less critical than in pediatric patients, attention to technical details is important also in adults, and Doppler parameters must be carefully adjusted to optimize detection of the small intratesticular vessels. Vascular findings within the torsed testis are related to the degree of torsion. High-grade torsions cause complete disappearance of flow signals from the testis, and color Doppler imaging may show only peritesticular vascularity (see **Fig. 2B**). In low-grade torsions (causing initially only obstruction of testicular veins), arterial signals may still be visible, although they are usually less numerous than within the contralateral asymptomatic testis (**Fig. 3**).[10] Color flow Doppler alone has a sensitivity of 86% to 94% and a specificity of 96% to 100% in diagnosing testicular torsion.[11,12] To reduce the number of false-negatives, the study must be completed with spectral analysis: waveforms evaluation of residual arterial flow in cases with low-grade torsion will show a high-resistance pattern, with an elevated resistivity index and

decreased or even reversed diastolic flow secondary to obstruction of venous outflow from the testis.[13,14] Once again, asymmetry of findings between the symptomatic and contralateral testis may help the diagnosis.

Torsion may be a transient and recurrent phenomenon. Patients with spontaneous detorsion of the torsed spermatic cord present with history of acute testicular pain followed by rapid disappearance of symptoms, and often report recurrent similar past episodes followed by asymptomatic periods. If the ultrasound study is performed shortly after the painful episode, postischemic testicular hyperemia may be observed and the gray-scale changes that ensued during the ischemic period may still be visible, with testicular enlargement and hypoechogenicity.[1,2] Clinical correlation helps avoid misinterpretation of these findings due to inflammation; proper recognition of torsion/detorsion syndrome is an indication for surgical exploration and testicular fixation to prevent recurrences. Furthermore, areas of focal infarction may develop during the ischemic episodes in these patients, usually presenting as

A

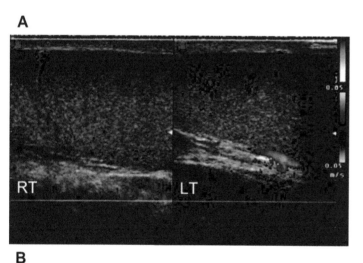

B

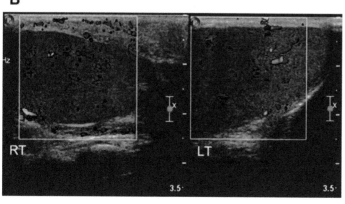

Fig. 3. Sagittal color Doppler images of the right (RT) and left (LT) testes in a 16-year-old boy with right-sided pain lasting 4 hours. (*A*) At admission, the right testis is slightly swollen, with normal echogenicity; a few flow signals are visible in it, but vascularity is markedly diminished compared with the left one. (*B*) The right testis could be salvaged at surgery and, at a follow-up evaluation 2 days later, intratesticular flow was visible and slightly increased compared with the left one. Thickening of the scrotal wall was also present.

hypoechoic, avascular, or hypovascular lesions, often with a wedge shape. If any doubts exist, unequivocal differentiation between hypovascular and avascular lesions can be obtained with contrast-enhanced ultrasonography.[15]

APPENDAGEAL TORSION

The testicular and epididymal appendages are remnants of the degenerating mesonephric and paramesonephric ducts. They are found, respectively, at the upper pole of the testis and the head of the epididymis. Both may be visible at ultrasound, especially when surrounded by a small quantity of fluid. The appendix testis is seen as an ovoid structure of up to 5 mm in the groove between the testis and the epididymis. It is isoechoic to the testis and occasionally may be cystic. The appendix epididymis is of the same approximate dimensions but is more often pedunculated.[15] These appendages may undergo torsion and, in children and young boys with acute scrotum, this is an important differential diagnosis. A firm diagnosis of appendageal torsion, in fact, allows for nonoperative management of the patient. Typically, on physical examination, a small, firm nodule is palpable on the superior aspect of the testis that exhibits a bluish discoloration through the overlying skin: the so-called blue dot sign. At ultrasonography, the testis has normal echotexture, and vascularization and the torsed appendix appears as a nodule of variable echogenicity adjacent to it. Reactive hydrocele, enlargement of the epididymal head, and skin thickening may be associated. The presence of a normal testis is the key differential feature from testicular torsion. On color Doppler imaging, the torsed appendix has no internal flow signals, whereas increased flow may be seen around it (**Fig. 4**).[16–18] A correlation seems to be apparent between the echogenicity of the torsed appendix and the time from beginning of symptoms. Park and coworkers[19] found that all torsed appendages were hypoechoic within 24 hours from onset of pain, whereas isoechogenic or hyperechogenic patterns were frequently observed in patients examined after 24 hours. This finding can possibly be explained by the development of necrotic and hemorrhagic changes within the torsed appendix over time. Furthermore, a manual detorsion maneuver had a higher success rate in hypoechoic appendages than in isoechogenic and hyperechoic ones.[20]

EPIDIDYMITIS AND ORCHITIS

Inflammatory conditions of the scrotum are the most frequent cause of acute scrotal pain in the

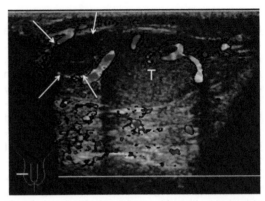

Fig. 4. Axial color Doppler evaluation of the right testis in a 3-year-old child with scrotal pain lasting 5 hours. The testis has normal shape, structure, and vascularization. The torsed testicular appendage (*arrows*) appears as a small hypoechoic avascular nodule surrounded by increased vascularity. T, testis.

adult population. The infection usually results from retrograde spread of urethral pathogens via the ejaculatory ducts and vas deferens; it first affects the tail of the epididymis and then extends to involve the body and head. Orchitis develops in 20% to 40% of cases through direct spread of infection. Sexually transmitted pathogens such as *Chlamydia trachomatis* and *Neisseria gonorrhea* are common in men younger than 35 years. In prepuberal boys and men older than 35 years, the disease is most frequently caused by *Escherichia coli* and *Proteus mirabilis*.[1,2,19,20] On gray-scale imaging, the involved portion of the epididymis is enlarged and hypoechoic. Hyperechogenic areas can be seen, and can be related to hemorrhagic changes. Thickening of the overlying scrotal wall and reactive hydrocele are usually associated. On color Doppler examination, increased blood flow to the enlarged epididymis is seen (**Fig. 5**). Because the presence of flow signals within the epididymis is a normal finding, comparison with the contralateral asymptomatic side may be useful. When the infection extends to the testis, orchitis is recognized by testicular enlargement, heterogeneously hypoechoic echostructure, and hyperemia on color Doppler imaging. With proper scanning technique, it is possible to demonstrate that, in these cases, intratesticular vessels have a normal, rectilinear course and, at spectral analysis, low-resistance waveforms, lower than in normal testes. Furthermore, intratesticular venous flow signals can be easily detected (**Fig. 6**).[1,2,21] In the proper clinical setting, this combination of findings indicates inflammatory disease. However, it must be underlined that focal intratesticular lesions with nodular shape may be encountered in

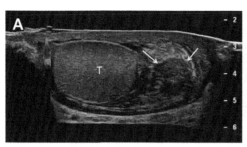 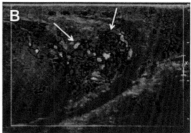

Fig. 5. (*A*) Extended-field-of-view sagittal image of the left hemiscrotum in a 37-year-old man with pain and tenderness. Enlargement and hypoechogenicity of the epididymal tail (*arrows*) is seen. (*B*) In the color Doppler image marked hypervascularity (*arrows*) is seen. T, testis. (*B*) Marked hypervascularity is seen.

orchitis, either because of focal inflammatory changes or, more frequently, heterogeneous appearance of diffuse disease. Although color Doppler imaging shows that most tumors have internal vessels with an irregular course, different from those observed in orchitis, this is not always the case, and focal testicular lesions should always be followed up until complete resolution occurs and is documented with ultrasound to rule out neoplastic disease. When infection is severe or goes untreated, epididymo-orchitis may be followed by complications such as pyocele, abscess formation, and testicular infarction. A pyocele, defined as presence of purulent fluid within the tunica vaginalis, develops when the mesothelial lining is breached and infection ensues in the cavity. At ultrasound, it can be recognized and differentiated from a hydrocele by the presence of thin septations and fine echogenic debris within the fluid.[1,2] Intraepididymal abscesses are easily recognized as hypoechoic areas, usually containing echogenic fluid, located within the involved portion of the epididymis and surrounded by increased vascular signals.[22] They have been found more commonly at the tail of the epididymis (**Fig. 7**). Intratesticular abscesses may be more difficult to diagnose because their appearance is more variable. They commonly appear as complex cystic lesions with irregular walls, low-level internal echoes, and hypervascular margins on color Doppler imaging; however, they may have a solid-like pattern, with mixed internal echogenicity and slightly hyperechoic borders.[23] Although these lesions show a lack of internal flow on color Doppler imaging,[24] confirmation of absence of vascularity with the use of contrast-enhanced ultrasonography may increase diagnostic confidence and allow them to be differentiated with certainty from poorly vascularized tumors (**Fig. 8**).[23] Although rarely, testicular infarctions may also develop as a complication of severe orchitis. In patients with severe edema, in fact, compression of testicular veins against the rigid tunica albuginea may ensue, resulting in venous infarction of the testis. Lesions may be either diffuse or focal and can be recognized by flow

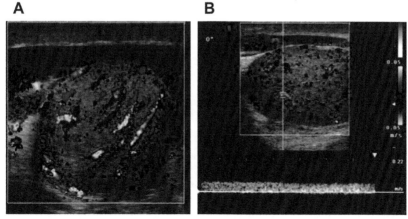

Fig. 6. Ultrasound Doppler study in a 70-year-old man with epididymo-orchitis presenting with pain and swollen right hemiscrotum. (*A*) Both the testis and epididymis are slightly enlarged and hypervascular, and a small amount of fluid is present with thin internal septa. (*B*). Intratesticular venous signals could be easily identified.

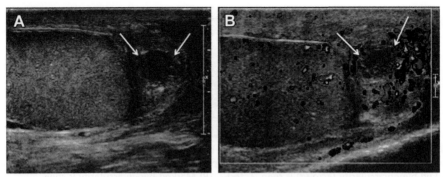

Fig. 7. Sagittal image of the epididymal tail in a 52-year-old man with epididymitis and epididymal abscess. (*A*) The abscess (*arrows*) is visible as a small collection containing hypoechogenic fluid. (*B*) On color Doppler imaging, the abscess (*arrows*) is surrounded by marked hypervascularity.

changes on Doppler examination, with complete absence of testicular flow or presence of areas of decreased vascularity. Waveform analysis can show intratesticular vessels with decreased or even reversed diastolic flow in these cases (**Fig. 9**). Contrast-enhanced ultrasound can also be useful in these patients to confirm the absence of vascularization within the affected areas.[23,25]

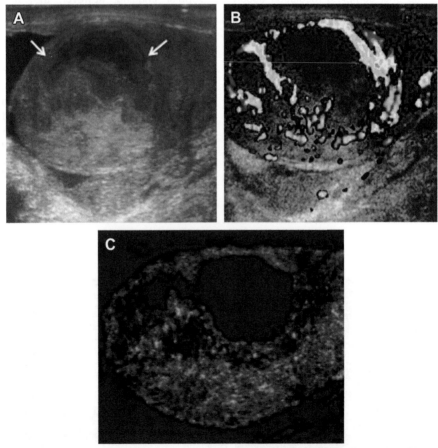

Fig. 8. Testicular abscess in a 47-year-old man with right testicular pain and fever. (*A*) Ultrasonography shows marked heterogeneity at the upper pole of the testis; a crescent-shaped hypoechoic area is visible in it (*arrows*). (*B*) Color Doppler image shows 2 ill-defined hypovascular zones surrounded by increased vascularity. (*C*) A contrast-enhanced ultrasound study allows precise delineation of the avascular necrotic area, which has an irregular shape and is smaller than that seen on color Doppler imaging.

A

B

C

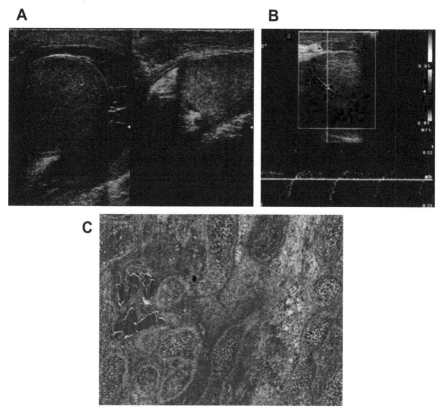

Fig. 9. (*A*) Composite axial image of the scrotum of a 58-year-old man with severe epididymo-orchitis. The right testis is swollen, hypoechoic, and surrounded by fluid, with many thin internal septations. (*B*) Only one vessel is visible within the testis, with reversed diastolic flow. (*C*) Histologic specimen from the testis shows edema, necrosis, and vascular congestion (hematoxylin eosin, original magnification ×10).

Less Common Causes of Acute Scrotum

Mumps orchitis

Orchitis is a well-known complication of mumps. It can be observed in approximately 18% of these patients, usually occurring within the first week after the parotid infection appears. However, orchitis may develop without parotid involvement. Clinically, testicular involvement is more commonly unilateral (70% of cases), with local inflammatory symptoms such as pain, tenderness, and scrotal redness. At ultrasonography, the involved testis appears inflamed: it is enlarged, with decreased echogenicity and increased vascularity on color Doppler imaging.[1,2,26] Mumps must be considered when these findings are not associated with signs of epididymitis. The most common pathologic type of mumps orchitis is the interstitial type, which is characterized by interstitial edema and mononuclear infiltration. Increased intratesticular pressure may lead to atrophy in 40% to 70% of cases, with possible development of sterility in 37% to 87%.[26]

Scrotal wall infections

Cellulitis of the scrotal wall is a common condition in patients who are obese, diabetic, or immunocompromised. Ultrasonography shows thickened scrotal wall, with increased blood flow seen on color Doppler imaging. Abscesses may develop, presenting as hypoechogenic areas with irregular walls and low-level internal echoes. Involvement of the scrotal wall may also be observed in patients with severe epididymo-orchitis, with spread of infection from the testis to the vaginalis cavity and scrotal wall (**Fig. 10**).

Fournier gangrene

Fournier gangrene is a potentially fatal polymicrobial necrotizing fasciitis of the perineum, perianal region, and scrotal wall in which infection induces an obliterative endarteritis, resulting in cutaneous and subcutaneous vascular necrosis. Diabetes mellitus and alcohol abuse are well-known predisposing factors. The diagnosis of Fournier gangrene is commonly made clinically, based on

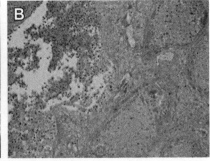

Fig. 10. (A) Axial image of the testis in a 65-year-old man with swollen scrotum, pain, and tenderness. The testis (T) is heterogeneous, with a fluid-filled abscess (*star*) in it; it is surrounded by echogenic fluid, and a breech (*open arrow*) is seen in the scrotal layers, with extension of infection into a subcutaneous abscess (*arrows*). (B) Histologic specimen from the testis showing an area of necrosis (hematoxylin eosin, original magnification ×20).

scrotal swelling, pain, hyperemia, pruritus, fever, and crepitus on palpation. Imaging is needed to confirm the diagnosis only in clinically ambiguous or questionable cases. At ultrasound, the scrotal and perineal walls are thickened and contain hyperechogenic foci that cast a posterior "dirty" shadow from reverberation artifacts arising from gas within the soft tissues (**Fig. 11**).[1,27] The testes and epididymi have a normal appearance and normal vascularization on color Doppler imaging, because blood supply to the scrotal wall is different from that to the testis. Although ultrasonography is able to diagnose the presence of a Fournier gangrene, computed tomography is the preferred imaging procedure in these patients, because it is able to assess the complete extent of subcutaneous emphysema, show the presence of fluid collections and abscesses, and recognize the spread of the disease process to the pelvis and retroperitoneum,[27] thus guiding surgical debridement of infected tissues.

Segmental testicular infarction

Segmental testicular infarction is a rare condition that presents with acute scrotal pain and is clinically indistinguishable from other causes of acute scrotum. Before the widespread use of imaging in acute testicular symptoms, it was commonly diagnosed only after orchidectomy. However, if a firm diagnosis of segmental testicular infarction is reached based on imaging appearances and negative tumor marker results, follow-up alone is now advocated, and surgery may be avoided.[28–31] Various pathologic conditions have been suggested as possible underlying causes of segmental testicular infarction, such as hypercoagulability disorders, vasculitis, torsion, trauma, infection, and iatrogenic vascular injury, but in many patients a cause is not found and the condition is termed *idiopathic*. Lesions seem more common at the upper pole of the testis, possibly because of the presence of vascular abnormalities at this site.[29] Furthermore, some authors[28–31] have

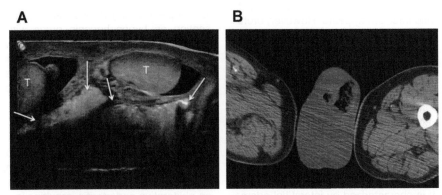

Fig. 11. (A) Axial extended-field-of-view ultrasound image in a 72-year-old man with diabetes with swollen and painful scrotum. Both testes (T) are normal, but diffuse thickening of the scrotal layers is present and, posteriorly to the testes, hyperechogenicity and reverberation artifacts from gas are seen (*arrows*). (B) Non–contrast-enhanced computed tomography image confirmed scrotal wall thickening and the presence of gas within scrotal soft tissues.

found this condition to be more frequent at the left testis, but data are conflicting about side prevalence. On ultrasonography, a typical segmental testicular infarct has been described as a solid and hypoechogenic area in the testis, oval- or wedge-shaped, with a lobular appearance. Multiple ischemic lobules can be seen in some cases, usually separated by an echogenic interface, often with vessels visible (**Fig. 12**). The infarcted areas may be almost isoechoic to the surrounding parenchyma (most frequent appearance in the early lesions), hypoechogenic, or mixed, and have absent or markedly diminished vascularity on color Doppler imaging (**Fig. 13**).[28–31] The differential diagnosis from a hypovascular tumor can be difficult if the infarct has a rounded shape and when vascularity is not completely absent. Contrast-enhanced ultrasonography can be used in these cases, because it allows better delineation of the morphologic features of this lesion, which are different from those of hypovascular tumors, and provides evidence of the ischemic nature of the disease process. When small vessels are still visible within the lesion, contrast-enhanced ultrasound can easily show that they are normal centripetal testicular arteries arising from the capsular vessels, and are not caused by tumor neovascularization.[31] Absence of intralesional flow and a perilesional rim of increased enhancement on contrast-enhanced magnetic resonance (MR) have been described as typical features in these cases.[29,30] Serial evaluation with contrast-enhanced ultrasound has shown that the latter of these findings is rare in lesions examined early (8% of cases), whereas it is commonly encountered (86%) on short-term follow-up studies (between 2 and 17 days).[31] Correlation with histology specimen in subacute infarctions suggests that perilesional rim enhancement may be caused by granulation tissue and neovasculature surrounding the infarcted lobules.[32] Decrease in size of the infarcted lobules and the reappearance of internal vascular signals are commonly found in long-term follow-up examinations, leading to almost disappearance of the lesions or late demonstration of a hypoechogenic triangular-shaped scar. The authors believe that, in clinical practice, when a segmental testicular infarction is

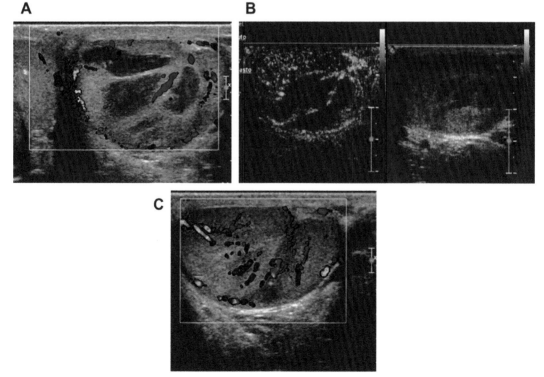

Fig. 12. (*A*) Axial color Doppler image in a 33-year-old man with acute pain in the left testis. Multiple areas with hypoechoic structure and lobular shape are seen, divided by echogenic septa within which some vessels are seen. (*B*) Contrast-enhanced ultrasound evaluation confirms that the lobules are avascular; they appear larger than in the color Doppler study. (*C*) Follow-up examination at 6 months shows scars within the testis, which is now homogeneously vascularized.

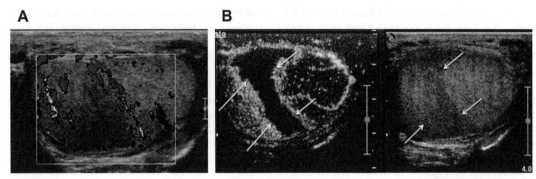

A   **B**

Fig. 13. (*A*) Sagittal scan of the right testis in a 47-year-old man with acute pain. A slightly hyperechoic triangular-shaped area is present without vascularity. (*B*) Contrast-enhanced ultrasound confirms avascularity in the affected area (*arrows*). Reduced, but still present, vascularization is appreciated at the lower pole of the testis.

suspected based on ultrasonographic and color Doppler findings, a contrast-enhanced examination (eg, MR imaging, ultrasound) is needed to rule out a hypovascular tumor, and then serial examinations with color Doppler imaging can be used to document healing of the disease process.

Schönlein-Henoch purpura
Schönlein-Henoch purpura is a systemic vasculitis that usually affects the skin, kidneys, gastrointestinal tract, and joints. It is more commonly encountered in the pediatric age group, and acute scrotal symptoms can be encountered in up to 15% of boys with this condition. The ultrasonographic findings include thickening of the scrotal skin, enlargement of the epididymis, and presence of a hydrocele. The testes are not affected, and present with normal volume, shape, and vasculature. The differential diagnosis from an episode of torsion is usually straightforward based on the latter finding.[33,34]

Acute idiopathic scrotal edema
Acute idiopathic scrotal edema is a frequent condition in boys (it is the fourth most common cause of acute scrotum after testicular torsion, torsion of testicular appendages, and infections) but is rare in adults. It is a self-limiting condition that usually resolves without sequelae in a few days. Clinically, it presents with scrotal enlargement, erythema, and, frequently, acute pain. Ultrasonography shows diffuse thickening and hypervascularity of the scrotal wall. The scrotal wall is easily compressible with the transducer, and involvement is usually bilateral. Both epididymi and testes are normal, with normal vascularization on color Doppler imaging. Thickening of the subcutaneous fat in the inguinal area and perineal region can be associated, and inguinal lymph nodes can be enlarged, with an oval shape and increased blood flow at their hilum.[35,36]

Scrotal hernia
A scrotal hernia may present as an acute mass in the groin and may be a cause of acute pain. The diagnosis is commonly based on physical examination, but ultrasonography may be requested in patients with equivocal findings. The ultrasonographic appearance depends on the contents within the hernial sac, usually intestinal loops (either small or large bowel or both) with associated portions of mesentery, and the omentum (**Fig. 14**). On ultrasound, the bowel loops can be collapsed, or fluid- or air-filled, whereas the presence of echogenic tissue indicates the presence of omental fat.[1] Peristaltic movements can be observed. The presence of dilated aperistaltic bowel loops must raise suspicion, in the proper clinical setting, of bowel strangulation.[37] Compression on the spermatic cord from a scrotal hernia may be the cause of testicular ischemia and can be detected on color Doppler ultrasonography.[38,39]

Spontaneous intratesticular hemorrhage
Spontaneous intratesticular hemorrhage is extremely rare, with no known risk factors. A report on the ultrasonographic findings for 2 patients with this condition described the presence of a heterogeneous intratesticular mass without internal vascular signal, even after ultrasound contrast injection (**Fig. 15**).[40] Orchidectomy was performed in both patients, because differentiating the lesions from a hypovascular tumor was deemed impossible. However, increasing experience with contrast-enhanced ultrasonography has shown that this technique is capable of differentiating hypovascular from truly avascular lesions. Based on this finding, a conservative approach now seems possible for all patients with focal testicular lesions that prove to be avascular after a contrast-enhanced ultrasound examination. A series of ultrasound examinations performed in the short term, and measurements of tumor markers, can

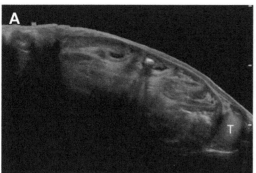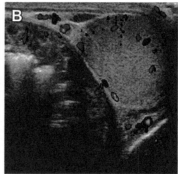

Fig. 14. (A) Extended-field-of-view ultrasound image of the right hemiscrotum in a patient with a large scrotal hernia and acute pain. The hernia contains bowel loops with air and the testis is displaced caudally. T, testis. (B) On color Doppler imaging, the testis appears somewhat compressed by the bowel, but has normal vascularization.

be used to monitor the disease process over time and guide therapeutic decisions.

Epididymal torsion

Isolated torsion of the epididymis is a rare cause of acute scrotum. A predisposing factor for this condition is the presence of a long and tortuous epididymis with a long mesorchium, or of epididymal-testicular dissociation. This condition presents with acute scrotal pain, which is difficult to differentiate from testicular or appendageal torsion on a clinical basis only. The ultrasonographic findings in one patient showed that the testis was normal, with regular vascularization, but that the epididymis was long and tortuous, was attached to the testis only at the level of the head, and had twisted on itself at the junction between the head and body. The epididymal body and tail were enlarged, almost avascular, with a heterogeneous echotexture. The epididymal head was markedly hypervascular, with vessels arranged in a whirling pattern at the point of torsion.[41]

Tension hydrocele

Hydrocele is one of the most common causes of scrotal swelling. It can be congenital (from a patent processus vaginalis); secondary to trauma, infection, or tumor; or idiopathic, related to increased serous fluid secretion or inadequate reabsorption of fluid in the vaginalis. Large and tense hydroceles can cause compression over the testis, producing morphologic and vascular changes. Increased intratesticular vascular resistances have been shown in patients with hydrocele, with return to normal values after hydrocelectomy.[42] Patients with testicular ischemia from large hydroceles seen on Doppler evaluation as markedly reduced intratesticular diastolic flow, or even as a lack of detectable flow signals, have been reported in the literature.[42–44] They presented clinically with severe pain, and it has been postulated that the association of pain and markedly reduced blood flow can classify the condition as a compartment syndrome within the tunica vaginalis.[43] Compression of the testis from the tense hydrocele may result in further

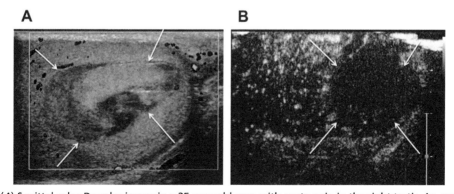

Fig. 15. (A) Sagittal color Doppler image in a 35-year-old man with acute pain in the right testis. An oval-shaped area is seen with a heterogeneous structure, both hyperechoic and hypoechoic (arrows). (B) The lesion was confirmed to be avascular using contrast-enhanced ultrasound (arrows). At surgery only hemorrhage was shown, and histologic examination of the testis confirmed hemorrhage without appreciable tumor.

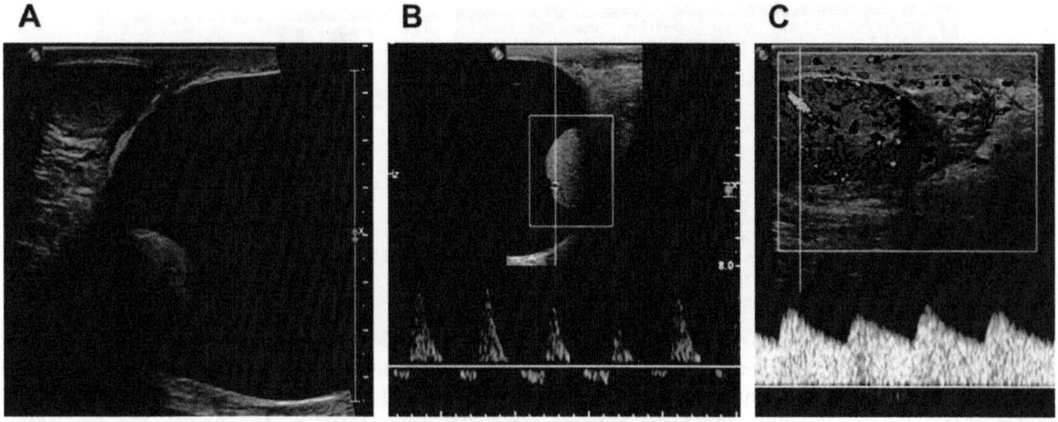

A **B** **C**

Fig. 16. (A) Axial ultrasound image in a 67-year-old man with a painful left-sided hydrocele. Both testes look normal, fluid within the hydrocele is anechoic, and the vaginalis surface is regular and smooth. (B) Color Doppler image shows reduced vascularity within the testis, and spectral analysis shows reversed diastolic flow. (C) Follow-up immediately after aspiration of 200 mL of serous fluid shows a hypervascular testis (a postischemic reaction), and spectral analysis shows both arterial and venous flow signals.

compromise of testicular viability, and no delay in treatment has been recommended (**Fig. 16**).[44]

NONSCROTAL CAUSES OF ACUTE SCROTUM

A variety of clinical problems that are not primarily caused by scrotal lesions may cause pain, enlargement, or changes of color of the scrotum, thus suggesting an acute scrotum. One of these clinical situations is frequent and well-known: patients with renal colic have pain that typically radiates to the testis. In this instance, patients may be encountered in whom flank pain is low or absent, who are referred for a scrotal ultrasound examination because clinical attention is given primarily to the testis. After a normal testicular study, careful interrogation is usually able to elicit a story of pain also at the flank, thus properly directing the examination toward the kidneys.

In addition, both intraperitoneal and retroperitoneal conditions can extend into the scrotum and suggest an acute situation. This event can occur from patency of the peritoneo-vaginalis foramen (especially in children) or from passage of fluid collections along the retroperitoneal spaces down to the perineal region, involving the scrotal wall. For instance, patients with appendicitis may have pus (or even the inflamed appendix) extending into the scrotum,[45,46] or patients with intraperitoneal hemorrhages can have blood that extends caudally and collects within the vaginalis.[47,48] Passage of fluid collection along the retroperitoneal fasciae is also possible[49,50] and, for instance, secondary scrotal involvement has been reported in neonates with spontaneous adrenal hemorrhages and after acute pancreatitis.

REFERENCES

1. Dogra V, Bhatt S. Acute painful scrotum. Radiol Clin North Am 2004;42:349–63.
2. Dogra VS, Gottlieb RH, Oka M, et al. Sonography of the scrotum. Radiology 2003;227:18–36.
3. Stavros T, Rapp C, McGrath J. Color duplex sonography of acute scrotal pain. In: Bluth EI, Arger PH, Benson CB, et al, editors. Ultrasound: a practical approach to clinical problems. New York: Thieme; 2000. p. 135–52.
4. Remer EM, Casalino DD, Arellano RS, et al. ACR appropriateness criteria: acute onset of scrotal pain - without trauma, without antecedent mass. Ultrasound Q 2012;28:47–51.
5. Piscaglia F, Nolsoe C, Dietrich C, et al. The EFSUMB guidelines and recommendations on the clinical practice of contrast-enhanced ultrasound (CEUS): update 2011 on non-hepatic applications. Ultraschall Med 2012;32:33–59.
6. Al-Salem AH. Intrauterine testicular torsion: a surgical emergency. J Pediatr Surg 2007;42:1887–91.
7. Sorensen MD, Galansky SH, Striegl AM, et al. Perinatal extravaginal torsion of the testis in the first month of life is a salvageable event. Urology 2003;62:132–4.
8. Zerin JM, DiPietro MA, Grignon A, et al. Testicular infarction in the newborn: ultrasound findings. Pediatr Radiol 1990;20:329–30.
9. Vijayaraghavan SB. Sonographic differential diagnosis of acute scrotum: real-time whirlpool sign, a key sign of torsion. J Ultrasound Med 2006;25: 563–74.
10. Cassar S, Bhatt S, Paltiel HJ, et al. Role of spectral Doppler sonography in the evaluation of partial testicular torsion. J Ultrasound Med 2008;27:1629–38.

11. Burks DD, Markey BJ, Burkhard TK, et al. Suspected testicular torsion and ischemia: evaluation with color Doppler sonography. Radiology 1990;175:815–21.

12. Yagil Y, Naroditsky I, Milhem J, et al. Role of Doppler ultrasonography in the triage of acute scrotum in the emergency department. J Ultrasound Med 2010;29: 11–21.

13. Lin EP, Bhatt S, Rubens DJ, et al. Testicular torsion: twists and turns. Semin Ultrasound CT MR 2007; 28:317–28.

14. Dogra VS, Sessions A, Mevorach RA, et al. Reversal of diastolic plateau in partial testicular torsion. J Clin Ultrasound 2001;29:105–8.

15. Valentino M, Bertolotto M, Derchi L, et al. Role of contrast enhanced ultrasound in acute scrotal diseases. Eur Radiol 2011;21:1831–40.

16. Sellars ME, Sidhu PS. Ultrasound appearances of the testicular appendages: pictorial review. Eur Radiol 2003;13:127–35.

17. Yang DM, Lim JW, Kim JE, et al. Torsed appendix testis: gray scale and color Doppler sonographic findings compared with normal appendix testis. J Ultrasound Med 2005;24:87–91.

18. Baldisserotto M, de Souza JC, Pertence AP, et al. Color Doppler sonography of normal and torsed testicular appendages in children. AJR Am J Roentgenol 2005;184:1287–92.

19. Park SJ, Kim HL, Yi BH. Sonography of intrascrotal appendage torsion: varying echogenicity of the torsed appendage according to the time from onset. J Ultrasound Med 2011;30:1391–6.

20. Garriga Farriol V, Pruna Comella X, Gallardo Agromayor E, et al. Gray-scale and power Doppler sonographic appearances of acute inflammatory diseases of the scrotum. J Clin Ultrasound 2000; 28:67–72.

21. Jee WH, Choe BY, Byun JY, et al. Resistive index of the intrascrotal artery in scrotal inflammatory disease. Acta Radiol 1997;38:1026–30.

22. Yang DM, Yoon MH, Kim HS, et al. Comparison of tuberculous and pyogenic epididymal abscesses: clinical, gray-scale sonographic, and color Doppler sonographic features. AJR Am J Roentgenol 2001;177:1131–5.

23. Lung PF, Jaffer OS, Sellars ME, et al. Contrast-enhanced ultrasound in the evaluation of focal testicular complications secondary to epididymitis. AJR Am J Roentgenol 2012;199:W345–54.

24. Dogra VS, Gottlieb RH, Rubens DJ, et al. Benign intratesticular cystic lesions: US features. Radiographics 2001;21:S273–81.

25. Yusuf G, Sellars ME, Kooiman GG, et al. Global testicular infarction in the presence of epididymitis: clinical features, appearances on grayscale, color Doppler and contrast-enhanced sonography and histologic correlation. J Ultrasound Med 2013;32: 175–80.

26. Basekim CC, Kizilkaya E, Pekkafali Z, et al. Mumps epididymo-orchitis: sonography and color Doppler sonographic findings. Abdom Imaging 2000;22: 322–5.

27. Levenson RB, Singh AK, Novelline RA. Fournier gangrene: role of imaging. Radiographics 2008; 28:519–28.

28. Bilagi P, Sriprasad S, Clarke J, et al. Clinical and ultrasound features of segmental testicular infarction: a six-years experience from a single center. Eur Radiol 2007;17:2810–8.

29. Fernandez-Perez GC, Tardaguila FM, Velasco M, et al. Radiologic findings of segmental testicular infarction. Am J Roentgenol 2005;184:1587–93.

30. Madaan S, Joniau S, Klockaerts K. Segmental testicular infarction: conservative management is feasible and safe. Eur Urol 2008;53:441–5.

31. Bertolotto M, Derchi LE, Sidhu PS, et al. Acute segmental testicular infarction at contrast-enhanced ultrasound: early features and changes during follow-up. AJR Am J Roentgenol 2011;196:834–41.

32. Aquino M, Nghiem H, Jafri SZ, et al. Segmental testicular infarction: sonographic findings and pathologic correlation. J Ultrasound Med 2013;32: 365–72.

33. Ben-Sira L, Laor T. Severe scrotal pain in boys with Henoch-Schönlein purpura: incidence and sonography. Pediatr Radiol 2000;30:125–8.

34. Sung EK, Setty BN, Castro-Aragon I. Sonography of the pediatric scrotum: emphasis on the Ts - torsion, trauma, and tumors. AJR Am J Roentgenol 2012;198:996–1003.

35. Lee A, Park SJ, Lee HK, et al. Acute idiopathic scrotal edema: ultrasonographic findings at an emergency unit. Eur Radiol 2009;19:2075–80.

36. Geiger J, Epelman M, Darge K. The fountain sign: a novel color Doppler sonographic finding for the diagnosis of acute idiopathic scrotal edema. J Ultrasound Med 2010;29:1233–7.

37. Subramanyam BR, Balthazar EJ, Raghavendra BN, et al. Sonographic diagnosis of scrotal hernia. AJR Am J Roentgenol 1982;139:535–8.

38. Eutermoser M, Nordenholz K. Testicular compromise due to inguinal hernia. West J Emerg Med 2012;13:131–2.

39. Desai Y, Tollefson B, Mills L, et al. Testicle ischemia resulting from a inguinal hernia. J Emerg Med 2012;43:e299–301.

40. Gaur S, Bhatt S, Derchi L, et al. Spontaneous intratesticular hemorrhage: two case descriptions and brief review of the literature. J Ultrasound Med 2011;30:101–4.

41. Dibilio D, Serafini G, Gandolfo NG, et al. Ultrasonographic findings of isolated torsion of the epididymis. J Ultrasound Med 2006;25:417–9.

42. Mihmanli I, Kantarci F, Kulaksizoglu H, et al. Testicular size and vascular resistance before and after

hydrocelectomy. AJR Am J Roentgenol 2004;183: 1379–85.

43. Douglas JW, Hicks JA, Manners J, et al. A pressing diagnosis – a compromised testicle secondary to compartment syndrome. Ann R Coll Surg Engl 2008;90:W6–8.

44. Wright LA, Gerscovich EO, Corwin MT, et al. Tension hydrocele: an additional cause of ischemia of the testis. J Ultrasound Med 2012; 31:2039–43.

45. Kynes JM, Rauth TP, McMorrow SP. Ruptured appendicitis presenting as acute scrotal swelling in a 23-month-old toddler. J Emerg Med 2012;43: 47–9.

46. Satchitananda K, Beese RC, Sidhu PS. Acute appendicitis presenting with a testicular mass:

ultrasound appearances. Br J Radiol 2000;73: 780–2.

47. Huckins DS, Barnett T. Occult splenic rupture presenting as acute scrotal swelling. J Emerg Med 2012;43:438–41.

48. Kwait DC, Nazarenko A, Derman A, et al. Perforated Meckel's diverticulum presenting as a hematocele on scrotal sonography. J Clin Ultrasound 2013;41:242–4.

49. Avolio L, Fusillo M, Ferrari G, et al. Neonatal adrenal hemorrhage manifesting as acute scrotum: timely diagnosis prevents unnecessary surgery. Urology 2002;59:601viii–x.

50. Kim SB, Je BK, Lee SH, et al. Scrotal swelling caused by acute necrotizing pancreatitis: CT diagnosis. Abdom Imaging 2011;36:218–21.

Postvasectomy Complications

Sadhna Verma, MD

KEYWORDS

- Vasectomy • Postvasectomy • Sperm granuloma • Closed-ended technique
- Open-ended technique • Scrotal pain • Spermatocele • Scrotal cellulitis

KEY POINTS

- Most vasectomy-related changes are attributable to chronic obstructive changes in the epididymis and vas deferens.
- Early complications such as hematomas and cellulitis/abscesses may occur, but are infrequent.
- Ultimately, it is useful to know the patient's vasectomy history when interpreting scrotal ultrasound. This information, along with an understanding of common postvasectomy changes, is vital for correct interpretation and proper management.

LEARNING OBJECTIVES

1. Review vasectomy procedure and types
2. Describe the normal physiologic changes following vasectomy
3. Review potential postvasectomy complications and illustrate the role of imaging in each

VASECTOMY

Vasectomy is currently the most effective available mode of male contraception. An estimated 40 to 60 million men worldwide rely on it, with slightly more than one-half million vasectomies being performed in the United States.[1] Reported rates of successful infertility for vasectomy exceed 98%.[2] As with any surgical procedure, certain complications and early/late changes may arise. However, before discussing such surgical complications, the types of procedures that may be used should be elaborated on.

VASECTOMY TECHNIQUES

There are 2 key surgical steps in performing vasectomy: (1) *isolation* of the vas deferens and (2) *occlusion* of the vas deferens. The risks of intra-operative and early postoperative pain, bleeding, and infection are related mainly to the method of vas isolation, whereas success/failure rates are primarily related to the method of vas occlusion. Methods of vas isolation include conventional vasectomy and minimally invasive vasectomy. Several studies have shown that minimally invasive vasectomy is superior to conventional vasectomy in several aspects, including patient discomfort during the procedure as well as fewer postoperative complications.[3] Both procedures are performed under local anesthesia.

Virtually all techniques of vasectomy use complete division of the vas with or without excision of a segment of the vas (**Fig. 1**). Following division, the divided vassal ends may be separated by one of several techniques and/or the flow of fluid and sperm with the vas lumen may be blocked by one of several methods. Per American Urological Association guidelines, 1 of 3 techniques of vas occlusion should be used. They include (1) cautery of the opened ends of the vas with subsequent interposition of the internal spermatic fascia between the 2 divided ends of the vas, (2) simple cautery of the opened ends of the vas without fascial interposition, or (3) an open-ended technique that uses leaving the divided testicular end of the vas unoccluded and subsequently using mucosal cautery on the abdominal end of the vas with superimposed fascial interposition.[3]

The hypothetical purpose of the open-ended technique is to (1) prevent or reduce

Department of Radiology, University of Cincinnati Medical Center, University of Cincinnati, ML 0761, 234 Goodman Street, Cincinatti, OH 45267-0761, USA

E-mail address: vermasm@ucmail.uc.edu

Ultrasound Clin 8 (2013) 545–550

http://dx.doi.org/10.1016/j.cult.2013.06.005

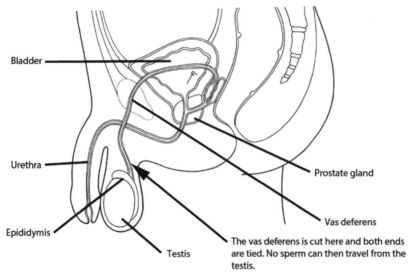

Bladder

Urethra

Epididymis

Testis

Prostate gland

Vas deferens

The vas deferens is cut here and both ends are tied. No sperm can then travel from the testis.

Fig. 1. Diagram detailing the close-ended technique. After the vas is exposed and occluded, a segment approximately 1 cm long is removed and the skin is sutured.

postvasectomy pain by decreasing back pressure from the epididymis[4] and (2) allow formation of a sperm granuloma at the transected testicular end of the vas, which some experts speculate might increase the chance of success of vasectomy reversal.[4,5]

POSTOPERATIVE COMPLICATIONS

A low frequency of complications is associated with vasectomy. The most important determinant of postoperative complications is operator experience. Surgeons performing more than 50 vasectomies a year had one-third the complication rate of those performing fewer than 10 procedures.[6]

Imaging complications can be divided into early, delayed, or late and are discussed as follows.

Early Complications and Changes

Postoperative bleeding and hematoma
Postoperative bleeding and hematoma formation is a complication of vasectomy (**Fig. 2**), with an incidence of about 2%.[6] The incidence of hematoma formation correlates with surgical experience. Minimally invasive vasectomies also demonstrate a lower incidence of hematomas given the minimal dissection required.[7] Painful

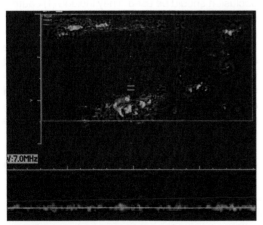

V:7.0MHz

Fig. 2. Sonographic image postvasectomy showing a fairly homogenous well-defined mass without internal flow, consistent with hematoma.

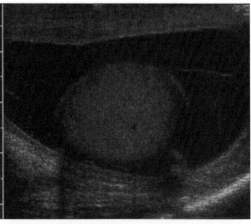

Fig. 3. Sonographic image of the testicle demonstrating a hypoechoic collection surrounding the testicle with multiple fine hyperechoic webs, most consistent with a hematocele given the patient's history of recent vasectomy.

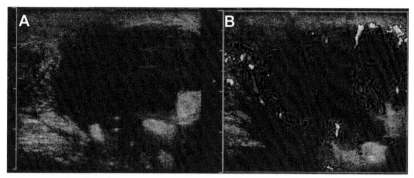

Fig. 4. (*A, B*) Sonographic images showing a heterogenous collection with associated adjacent inflammatory changes. These findings are consistent with postoperative cellulitis and abscess formation.

scrotal swelling is a typical chief complaint in affected patients. Sonographic features include a heterogeneous fluid collection adjacent to the testicle, which shows no internal Doppler flow.

Hematocele

A hematocele is an accumulation of blood within the tunica vaginalis that may be acute or chronic. Although vasectomy is a known cause, it is relatively uncommon. Other possible causes include trauma, torsion, and testicular tumors. Initially, an early hematocele is slightly echogenic. Its appearance becomes more complex over time, with septa, fluid-fluid levels, and echogenic debris (Fig. 3). Chronicity is indicated by the development of a heterogeneous capsule, which may calcify and create mass effect over the contour of the testis. Most hematoceles resolve with conservative therapy, although chronic complex hematoceles may require surgical management.[8]

Cellulitis/abscess

Infection is also a possible complication after vasectomy. The incidence has dramatically decreased over the past few decades, declining from 12% to 38% to around 1% to 2% based on surgical experience and refinement of technique.[3,9] Unfortunately, there have been 4 cases of Fournier's gangrene reported as well as 7 cases of coagulase-negative staphylococcal endocarditis.[10] More typically, cellulitis and/or abscess formation may be visible on ultrasound as a heterogeneously echogenic fluid collection with adjacent inflammatory changes (Fig. 4A). The periphery of the abscess may be hyperemic on Doppler interrogation (see Fig. 4B).

POSTOPERATIVE CHANGES
Tubular Ectasia of the Epididymis

The passage of sperm into an obstructed epididymis and vas deferens after vasectomy results in increased intraluminal pressure within the epididymis. This obstruction results in congestion and subsequent dilatation of the efferent ductules. Fluid absorption within the ductules then increases, and the normal columnar ciliated cells of the ductules disappear.[11] On sonography, this presents as thickening and distension of the epididymis with a finely speckled appearance (Fig. 5A)

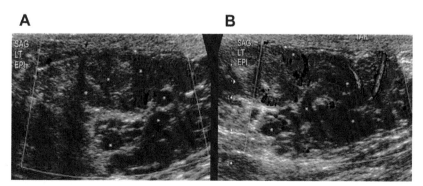

Fig. 5. (*A, B*) Sonographic images from different patients, which show dilated tubules (*asterisk*) near the mediastinum testis with no flow on Doppler evaluation. Although this finding can be seen with other causes of vas deferens obstruction, a small study showed 21 of 24 patients with tubular ectasia had a history of vasectomy.[3] Differential diagnosis includes intratesticular varicocele and malignancy.

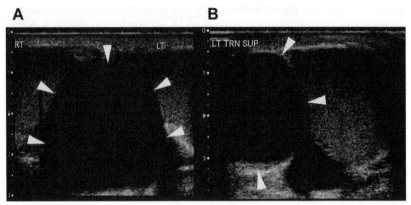

Fig. 6. (*A*, *B*) Sonographic images from different patients show a hypoechoic mass (*arrowheads*) containing speckled internal echoes. This appearance has been termed the "Falling snow sign" and is the result of movement of spermatozoa within the cyst. These are often associated with ductal ectasia.

without Doppler flow on interrogation (see **Fig. 5B**). The vas deferens may also be thickened. It is important to realize that other causes of vas deferens obstruction can result in this appearance; however, one study suggests that this appearance is highly suggestive of a postvasectomy testicle.[12] In addition, it is important to realize that this entity is separate from tubular ectasia of the rete testis, which represents dilatation of the tubules in the testis itself. However, this entity is also associated with conditions causing epididymal or efferent duct obstruction such as vasectomy.[11] Malignancy can also cause this appearance, particularly epididymal cystadenomas or any other tumor that may cause epididymal or vas deferens obstruction.

Late Changes

Spermatoceles
Spermatoceles are cystic structures filled with milky fluid containing sperm, lymphocytes, and cellular debris that result from the chronic obstruction and dilatation of the efferent tubules. Spermatoceles are typically seen in association with tubular ectasia of the epididymis.[13] Tubular ectasia of the epididymis appear as multichambered anechoic cysts in the epididymis or cystic lesions with low-level echoes (**Fig. 6**). When spermatoceles are anechoic, they are indistinguishable from an epididymal cyst. In a series by Holden and List,[14] epididymal cysts were more common in the general population (75% of lesions); however, in postvasectomy patients spermatoceles were more likely. When internal echoes are present, a technique using the mechanical properties of color Doppler may help confirm that a lesion represents a spermatocele. When color Doppler is applied over a spermatocele, the internal echoes within the spermatocele move away from the

transducer, giving an appearance similar to falling snow.[15]

Sperm granuloma
Sperm granuloma formation is a late finding following vasectomy that occurs in up to 40% of patients; however, very few of these patients experience pain. Sperm granulomas form as a granulomatous reaction following extravasation of sperm into the walls and interstitium of the epididymis and vas deferens (**Fig. 7**).[16] This entity is also along the spectrum of tubular ectasia of the epididymis. The presence of chronically increased pressures can no longer be compensated by cystic dilatation of the efferent ductules. It is thought that granuloma formation may help vent high intraepididymal pressures.[17]

Sperm granulomas are typically well-circumscribed, hypoechoic, and heterogeneous lesions

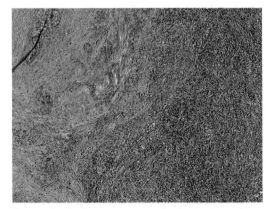

Fig. 7. Histologic appearance of a sperm granuloma. Vas deferens lumen is noted on the upper left; an intense inflammatory reaction is seen on the right.

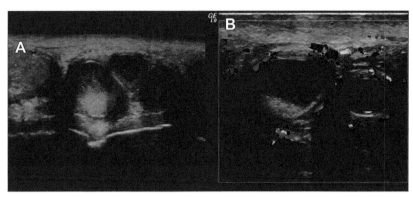

Fig. 8. (*A, B*) Sonographic images (*A*) from a patient status postvasectomy showing multiple hypoechoic extratesticular masses, consistent with sperm granulomas. (*B*) Doppler evaluation shows the masses are not hypervascular.

found within the epididymis, which may or may not show hypervascularity (**Fig. 8**).[18] Calcification occurs in approximately 10% of cases. Adenomatoid tumors may have a similar appearance; however, knowing the patient's vasectomy history aids in narrowing the diagnosis (**Fig. 9**A, B).

Other vasectomy-related findings
Many other benign lesions may be seen on ultrasound after vasectomy and include varicoceles, hydroceles, epididymal cysts, and testicular cysts. However, these abnormalities occur at a similar frequency to patients with or without a prior vasectomy.[11] Patients may also present with postvasectomy pain syndrome with scrotal pain unilaterally or bilaterally. The pathogenesis of pain in these patients is poorly understood but various mechanisms have been postulated including epididymal congestion, perineural fibrosis, extravasation of sperm, vascular stasis, painful sperm granulomas, lack of sperm granulomas (due to their inherent nature to relieve proximal obstruction and decompress the epididymis and vas), and circulating anti-sperm antibodies.[2,19–21]

SUMMARY

Most vasectomy-related changes are attributable to chronic obstructive changes in the epididymis and vas deferens. Early complications such as hematomas and cellulitis/abscesses may occur, but are infrequent. Ultimately, it is useful to know the patient's vasectomy history when interpreting scrotal ultrasound. This information, along with an understanding of common postvasectomy changes, is vital for correct interpretation and proper management.

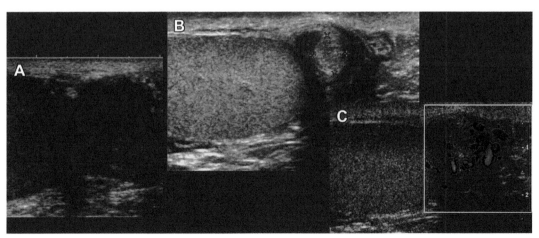

Fig. 9. (*A–C*) Sonographic images (*A*) from a 41 year old with a testicular lump shows a slightly hypoechoic mass in the tail of the epididymis originally reported as concerning for an adenomatoid tumor; cytologic correlation was recommended. Instead, close sonographic follow-up was performed. On follow-up (*B, C*) the mass was slightly smaller and more hyperechoic. Given the recent history of vasectomy, these findings were more consistent with a sperm granuloma.

REFERENCES

1. Peterson HB, Curtis KM. Clinical practice. Long-acting methods of contraception. N Engl J Med 2005;353(20):2169–75.
2. Schwingl PJ, Guess HA. Safety and effectiveness of vasectomy. Fertil Steril 2000;73(5):923–36.
3. Sharlip ID, Belker AM, Honig S, et al. Vasectomy: AUA guideline. J Urol 2012;188(Suppl 6):2482–91.
4. Shapiro EI, Silber SJ. Open-ended vasectomy, sperm granuloma, and postvasectomy orchialgia. Fertil Steril 1979;32(5):546–50.
5. Errey BB, Edwards IS. Open-ended vasectomy: an assessment. Fertil Steril 1986;45(6):843–6.
6. Kendrick JS, Gonzales B, Huber DH, et al. Complications of vasectomies in the United States. J Fam Pract 1987;25(3):245–8.
7. Sokal D, McMullen S, Gates D, et al. A comparative study of the no scalpel and standard incision approaches to vasectomy in 5 countries. The Male Sterilization Investigator Team. J Urol 1999;162(5):1621–5.
8. Garriga V, Serrano A, Marin A, et al. US of the tunica vaginalis testis: anatomic relationships and pathologic conditions. Radiographics 2009;29(7):2017–32.
9. Randall PE, Ganguli L, Marcuson RW. Wound infection following vasectomy. Br J Urol 1983;55(5):564–7.
10. Awsare NS, Krishnan J, Boustead GB, et al. Complications of vasectomy. Ann R Coll Surg Engl 2005;87(6):406–10.
11. Reddy NM, Gerscovich EO, Jain KA, et al. Vasectomy-related changes on sonographic examination of the scrotum. J Clin Ultrasound 2004;32(8):394–8.
12. Ishigami K, Abu-Yousef MM, El-Zein Y. Tubular ectasia of the epididymis: a sign of postvasectomy status. J Clin Ultrasound 2005;33(9):447–51.
13. Woodward PJ, Schwab CM, Sesterhenn IA. From the archives of the AFIP: extratesticular scrotal masses: radiologic-pathologic correlation. Radiographics 2003;23(1):215–40.
14. Holden A, List A. Extratesticular lesions: a radiological and pathological correlation. Australas Radiol 1994;38(2):99–105.
15. Sista AK, Filly RA. Color Doppler sonography in evaluation of spermatoceles: the "falling snow" sign. J Ultrasound Med 2008;27(1):141–3.
16. Lee JC, Bhatt S, Dogra VS. Imaging of the epididymis. Ultrasound Q 2008;24(1):3–16.
17. Jarvis LJ, Dubbins PA. Changes in the epididymis after vasectomy: sonographic findings. AJR Am J Roentgenol 1989;152(3):531–4.
18. Kumar A, Aggarwal S. Atypical sperm granuloma of the epididymis mimicking a testicular mass. Can Assoc Radiol J 1993;44(2):135–7.
19. Balogh K, Argenyi ZB. Vasitis nodosa and spermatic granuloma of the skin: an histologic study of a rare complication of vasectomy. J Cutan Pathol 1985;12:528.
20. Tandon S, Sabanegh E Jr. Chronic pain after vasectomy: a diagnostic and treatment dilemma. BJU Int 2008;102:166.
21. Christiansen CG, Sandlow JI. Testicular pain following vasectomy: a review of postvasectomy pain syndrome. J Androl 2003;24:293.

Ultrasound Elastography of the Kidney

Nicolas Grenier, MD[a,b,*], Jean-Luc Gennisson, PhD[c],
François Cornelis, MD[a], Yann Le Bras, MD[a],
Lionel Couzi, MD, PhD[b,d]

KEYWORDS

- Renal elasticity • Elastography • Supersonic shearwave imaging • ARFI • Renal transplant

KEY POINTS

- Quantification of tissue stiffness using ultrasound is more complex within the kidney than within the liver.
- Due to compartmentalization and high tissue heterogeneities, sonography-guided techniques seem more appropriate.
- Variability of measurements is increased by the risks of applied transducer pressure on abdominal wall and to tissue anisotropy.
- More experience is needed in preclinical models and in patient cohorts with pathologic correlation to understand better which are the physical factors of variation and the histopathologic causes of elasticity changes.
- Noninvasive imaging could participate in this challenge in the near future using functional, structural, or molecular approaches.

INTRODUCTION

Until now, imaging of the kidney has been based mainly on morphologic evaluation the parenchyma, excretory system, and intrarenal vasculature using ultrasound sonography (US) and Doppler, computed tomography, and magnetic resonance (MR) imaging. Functional parameters become now more and more accessible with MR imaging, such as perfusion, filtration, and diffusion measurements. However, structural assessment of the renal parenchyma remains a challenge. Among imaging methods used for that purpose, elastography is an attractive technique that has already been demonstrated in the liver.[1–3] Although US elastography has gained experience and validation in clinical practice for estimation of liver tissue changes related to fibrosis or steatohepatitis, little has been done now to evaluate its potential role for renal tissue changes.

As in the liver, the main factor of chronic renal function alteration is related to progressive changes of extracellular matrix leading to progression of fibrosis. This process, called chronic kidney disease (CKD), shows an increased incidence and prevalence in developed countries, particularly in

Disclosures of Potential Conflicts of Interest: N. Grenier is a member of the scientific advisory board of Super-Sonic Imagine. J.L. Gennisson is a consultant for SuperSonic Imagine.
F. Cornelis, Y. Le Bras, and L. Couzi have no conflicting financial interests.
[a] Service d'Imagerie Diagnostique et Interventionnelle de l'Adulte, Groupe Hospitalier Pellegrin, CHU de Bordeaux, Place Amélie Raba-Léon, Bordeaux Cedex 33076, France; [b] Radiology Department, Université Bordeaux Segalen, Bordeaux, France; [c] Institut Langevin – Ondes et Images, ESPCI ParisTech, CNRS UMR7587, INSERM U979, ESPCI, 10 rue Vauquelin, Paris 75005, France; [d] Nephrology Department, Service de Néphrologie et Transplantation Rénale, Groupe Hospitalier Pellegrin, CHU de Bordeaux, Place Amélie Raba-Léon, Bordeaux Cedex 33076, France
* Corresponding author. Service d'Imagerie Diagnostique et Interventionnelle de l'Adulte, Groupe Hospitalier Pellegrin, CHU de Bordeaux, Place Amélie Raba-Léon, Bordeaux Cedex 33076, France.
E-mail address: nicolas.grenier@chu-bordeaux.fr

the context of diabetes and hypertension-related nephropathies.[4] It causes end-stage renal failure, with its extensive morbidity and mortality and increases health costs. In most types of kidney diseases, CKD progression is characterized by progressive fibrotic processes that may involve first either glomeruli (glomerulosclerosis) or the interstitial space (interstitial fibrosis), depending on the initial nephropathy.[5,6] Similarly, in renal transplantation, the development of interstitial fibrosis and tubular atrophy (IF/TA), previously called chronic allograft nephropathy,[7,8] is the major determinant of renal allograft failure.

Because it is a progressive process, CKD justifies developing more efficient diagnostic strategies by using noninvasive methods. These new approaches require defining and validating adequate imaging biomarkers, with their intrinsic variability and interoperator reproducibility before being used in clinical practice. Diffusion-weighted MR imaging was recently proposed in experimental interstitial renal fibrosis[9] but no clinical validation has been reported yet. Application of US elastography to the kidney has been shown to be possible and the first results are encouraging. However, the kidney is a much more complex organ than the liver, with 2 anatomic compartments, cortex and medulla, a high vascularity, and a urinary excretion function. Therefore, all these parameters must be taken into account to understand better the intrinsic and extrinsic factors of variation on elasticity measurements before extending this method to large clinical trials.

The purposes of this review are to expose the main results, advantages, and limitations of US elastography for quantifying chronic degenerative processes in renal diseases and to propose new fields of application.

TECHNIQUES OF US ELASTOGRAPHY

Elastography techniques presented in this article can be classified into 2 main categories: the quasi-static techniques and the dynamic techniques. The difference between these 2 categories is very important because they do not provide the same information on mechanical parameters. Quasi-static elastography provides a strain image of the investigated organ, proportional to elasticity, then qualitative, whereas dynamic elastography provides a quantitative image or only one quantitative value of elasticity. Both techniques and their variants are explained in the following:

- Quasi-static elastography, also called by manufacturers "real-time elastography," was the first elastography technique, developed by the Ophir group at the beginning of the 1990s.[10] This technique is simple to implement and is widespread in the world of radiology. This technique is based on a quasi-static deformation or strain (ε) of the medium. Hence strain is related to the elasticity defined by the Young's modulus (E), through the Hooke's law (Eqn. 1), and the quantification of the deformation can provide a qualitative estimation of the Young's modulus.

$$E = \frac{\sigma}{\varepsilon} \qquad (1)$$

where σ is the stress applied to the medium, but which is never quantified.

To recover strain, 2 images are extracted before and after compression of the tissue (**Fig. 1**). Strain maps are then calculated from both images by spatial derivation following one or possibly 2 directions for the most evolved approaches. Most

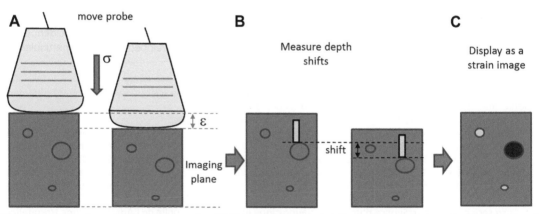

Fig. 1. Principle of quasi-static elastography. (*A*) The probe is placed at the surface of the investigated organ and small compression is applied. Images are acquired before and after compression. (*B*) By taking small windows within the image of raw US signals, a displacement shift in depth is recovered. (*C*) Then, by calculating the derivative of the displacement, the final strain image is obtained and displayed.

often, the displacement, which is relatively large, is calculated by a 2D correlation of B-mode images. The main limits of this technique are the control of the applied strain, which remains operator dependent, and the absence of a specific quantification. In addition, the use of a strain applied by the operator limits the technique to superficial organs, mainly the breast or the thyroid.

- Dynamic elastography is based on the propagation of mechanical or elastic waves in the body. In a quasi-incompressible medium such as the human body, the human body is almost constituted of 75% of water, which is an incompressible material; the Young's modulus is directly related to the speed (V_S) of a kind of elastic waves, the shear waves, where ρ is the density about 1000 kg m^{-3} (Eqn. 2):

$$E = 3\rho V_S^2 \qquad (2)$$

By generating a shear wave within the tissues using an external source (in this article a low-frequency vibrator or US radiation force) and by using 1D or 2D US to follow their propagation, dynamic elastography can then retrieve a quantitative value of the Young's modulus by estimating the speed of the shear waves. In this article, 3 dynamic elastography methods are developed: Fibroscan-transient elastography, Acoustic Radiation Force Impulse–Shear Wave Speed (ARFI-SWS), and Supersonic Shear wave Imaging (SSI).

- Fibroscan-transient elastography, originally called the "shear elasticity probe," was the first quantitative elastography method available on the market. It comes from the

Langevin Institute at the end of the 1990s.[11,12] It is a 1D US method based on a low-frequency (50 Hz) transient pulse transmitted in the medium and a recording of the propagating shear wave by using one single US transducer (5 MHz). First, the piston through the front face of the transducer will give a slight pulse on the medium, which generates a spherical compression wave as well as a shear wave (**Fig. 2**). The displacement generated, which is a function of depth and of time, is thus estimated by correlations of retro-diffused echoes (via US "speckle") at a frame rate of more than a thousand times per second. This device was the first to use the principle of ultrafast imaging in 1D to visualize in a transitory manner the propagation of shear waves. Then, by measuring the shear wave phase at each depth, the phase velocity of the shear wave at the central frequency is calculated in a given window of depth (from 20 to 60 mm). By considering also the medium as homogeneous and nonviscous, the elasticity of the medium is retrieved by using Eqn. 2.

- The concept of quantitative ARFI-SWS[13] is based on the use of the US radiation pressure as a shear-wave source. When USs are focused during a long period of time (hundreds of μs vs 1–10 μs for classical US B-mode), a force, called US radiation pressure, is generated at the focal spot. This force pushes tissues along the US axis like a US wind. As biologic tissues are elastic, after the force application, they come back to their original position, inducing a local vibration generating shear waves. Then shear waves

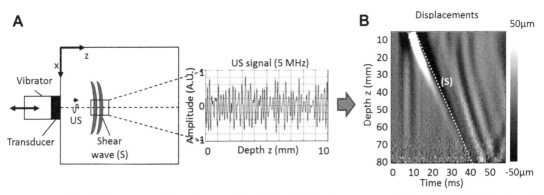

Fig. 2. Principle of Fibroscan-transient elastography. (*A*) A slight low-frequency pulse (typically 50 Hz) is given at the surface of the investigated medium with the front face of the transducer working in emission-reception at a high frame rate (some kHz). This pulse induces the propagation of shear waves, which induces movement within the raw frequency US signal recorded. (*B*) By cross-correlating the acquired signals, a displacements map showing shear-wave propagation in depth as a function of time is calculated. The shear-wave speed is then recovered by the estimating the slope of the shear wave.

are locally followed using US with a high frame rate (several kHz) closely to the source (some millimeters). Last, by using a time-of-flight algorithm, the shear-wave velocity is retrieved. In this technique measurements are provided on a small window placed at the wanted depth within organs. US devices using this method act as a 1D technique for elasticity measurement, but using a 2D US image (B-mode) to position the estimation box at the desire location within the organ (**Fig. 3**). Thus it needs several measurements and a longer time of acquisition to retrieve elasticity of a whole organ.

- The heart of the SSI technique is described by 2 fundamental concepts, the association of the acoustic radiation force (US radiation pressure) to generate a Mach cone and the US ultrafast imaging technique.[14] This technique, originally developed at the Langevin Institute, uses several successive focalized US spots at different depths (classically 4–5 spots) to illuminate a large part of the medium at one time. The different spherical waves generated for each radiation pressure spot interfere in a Mach cone in which the source propagates faster than the generated shear wave, creating a quasi-plane shear-wave front in the imaging plane (cylindrical in 3 dimensions) (**Fig. 4**). This constructive phenomenon increases the amplitude of the wave and thus the signal-to-noise ratio of the displacement field. Finally, only one Mach cone makes it possible to illuminate almost all the medium with one quasi-plane shear wave. Then ultrafast US imaging makes it possible to sound the entire imaging plane with a very high temporal resolution in one single acquisition, typically at a frame rate of 5000 images per second. Therefore, there is no need to stroboscope the acquisition several times to acquire an entire shear-wave field, allowing the creation of real-time images by carrying out the entire shear-wave field in less than 30 ms, which facilitates the examination, and fast averaging of acquired images to increase robustness.

TECHNICAL IMPACT ON RENAL SAMPLING

The quasi-static elastography technique is inadequate for renal purposes because the kidneys are deep and because they do not provide quantitative data.[15,16] Dynamic elastography techniques based on shear-wave propagation are more appropriate.

Among these techniques, the Fibroscan elastography system is also inappropriate for the kidney for several reasons: (1) first, there is no B-mode control and, as the sample volume is fixed

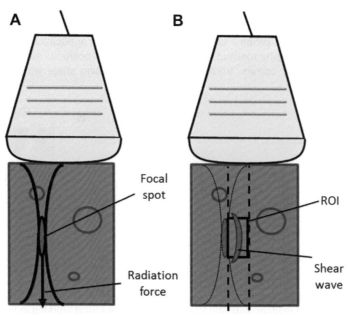

Fig. 3. Principle of ARFI. (*A*) A radiation force is created from a focal spot within the organ by focusing US, creating a local shear-wave source that is propagated perpendicularly to the US axis. (*B*) On a few transducers close to the focal spot, the displacements of the shear wave are recovered, allowing a 1D measurement of shear elasticity in the region-of-interest (ROI).

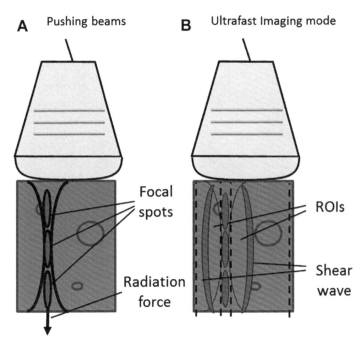

Fig. 4. Principle of SSI. (*A*) Multiple focal spots are created in depth along the same axis, generating a Mach cone acting as a shear-wave source. (*B*) By using an ultrafast imaging mode, the propagating shear wave is caught in the entire field of imaging, allowing the reconstruction of a 2D elasticity map.

in depth and size, it is extremely difficult and hazardous to position adequately the sample volume on the renal parenchyma, which is located at a variable depth and, moreover, to focus sampling on the cortex versus medulla. A manual adjustment could be considered in transplanted kidneys, because it is more superficially located, but it stays hazardous without real-time US control; moreover, such adjustment would require the pressure put on the probe to be modified, which would change elasticity values; (2) second, the mechanical wave must be applied on a rigid surface, such as the rib cage, to avoid compression effects by the probe, which is impossible for the kidney. Despite these limitations, Fibroscan transient elastography was used in 2 recent series of transplanted kidneys.[17,18] The latter reported that body mass index, skin-allograft distance, and perirenal or intrarenal fluid accumulation were important confounders of successful kidney stiffness measurements. The same authors mentioned that the heterogeneous renal morphology and several technical confounding factors negatively affect measurability of elasticity by this technique. Further technical modifications were called to improve its applicability for kidney assessment.

The ARFI system is more appropriate because it is US-guided, allowing a sample volume to be positioned in depth and to sample cortex and medulla selectively. It provides a monodimensional

real-time sampling (**Fig. 5**) or a fixed bidimensional quantitative mapping.

The SSI technique provides a real-time bidimensional quantitative mapping and is implemented on low-frequency curved arrays, for native and deep transplanted kidneys, and on high-frequency linear arrays, for superficial transplanted kidneys (**Fig. 6**).

IMPACT OF RENAL CHARACTERISTICS ON ELASTICITY VALUES

Measuring shear-wave velocity within the kidney with any of these systems must be performed with caution because of the sensitivity to many mechanical parameters, such as anisotropy and vascularization. A clear assessment of these factors of variation is essential to decrease the intrinsic variability of in vivo measurements, and to increase the reproducibility of the method. These factors are compressibility of renal transplants, anisotropy of renal architecture, high degree of renal vascularity, and possible increase of urinary pressure:

- Whereas native kidneys are quite deep within the abdomen and hardly compressible, renal transplants are more superficially located in the iliac fossa. For this reason, a manual compression of renal parenchyma by the

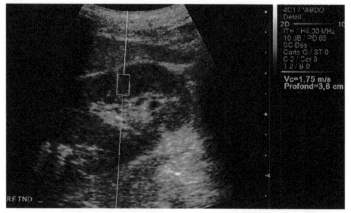

Fig. 5. Example of intrarenal shear-wave velocity measurement with the ARFI technique.

US probe is possible during scanning. The same phenomenon is observed on the liver parenchyma with higher elasticity values on the left lobe, using a compliant epigastric window, than on the right lobe, using a rigid intercostal window. For this reason, Syversveen and colleagues[19] evaluated, quantitatively, the effect of probe compression on elasticity values, using a mechanical device and calibrated compression forces with ARFI on the renal cortex of 31 kidney transplants. Comparison showed highly significant differences of mean shear-wave velocity between the 5 different compression weights (**Fig. 7**).

- In the kidney, the intrinsic architecture of the parenchyma is highly oriented, or anisotropic: Henle loops and vasa recta within medulla and the collecting ducts within cortex and medulla are parallel and oriented from the capsule to the papilla within each renal segment. Using MR imaging, the degree of anisotropy has been estimated to be around 15% in the cortex and 30% in the medulla.[20] For this reason, the authors evaluated in vivo the effect of intrarenal anisotropy on elasticity values in 6 pig kidneys, scanned peroperatively.[21] To evaluate this impact of anisotropy, acquisitions were performed in a renal segment with a pyramid axis parallel to US

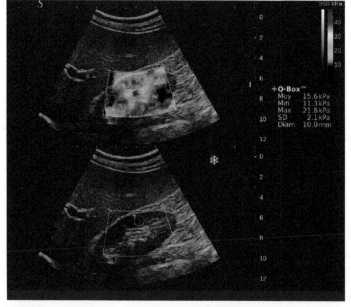

Fig. 6. Example of elasticity mapping in a native kidney with the SSI technique.

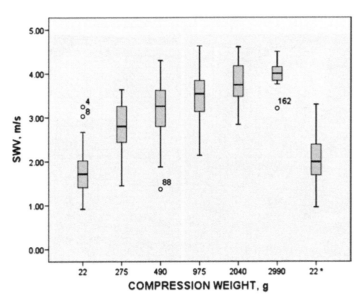

Fig. 7. Effect of probe compression. Box-and-whiskers plot of shear-wave velocities (SWV) by increasing compression weights and return to very light compression, using the ARFI technique. *, 22 g compression after removing higher compression weight. (*From* Syversveen T, Midtvedt K, Berstad AE, et al. Tissue elasticity estimated by acoustic radiation force impulse quantification depends on the applied transducer force: an experimental study in kidney transplant patients. Eur Radiol 2012;22:2134; with permission.)

beam, then in a renal segment with a pyramid axis perpendicular to the US beam. When emission of the US beam is sent parallel to renal microstructures, the shear wave propagates perpendicular to these, creating multiple vascular and tubular interfaces, thus decreasing its speed of propagation and resulting in lower elasticity values. Conversely, when emission of the US beam is sent perpendicular to these structures, the shear wave propagates at a higher speed, without interfaces, resulting in higher elasticity values (**Fig. 8**). The mean variation of the shear modulus due to anisotropy was 10.5% in the outer cortex, 29.7% in the inner cortex, and 31.8% in the medulla in normal conditions. Therefore, when performing renal US elastography, a clear identification of sampled renal segments and their orientation according to the US beam is mandatory, which is of prime importance for interpatient comparisons and longitudinal follow-up.

• The kidney is highly vascularized, mainly the cortex, with an eighth of the cardiac blood flow being distributed into each kidney. The degree of vascular pressure also influences elasticity values. In the same study, a significant decrease of elasticity was noted after ligation of the renal artery, this effect predominating within the cortex (**Fig. 9**).[21] Central regions of the kidney are less sensitive to

changes in renal perfusion pressure, because medullary blood pressure and flow are lower at baseline. Decrease of elasticity during ischemia was already observed using MR elastography, whereby cortical and medulla stiffness changed by ~30% and ~20%, respectively.[22] Conversely, in the authors' pig study, a huge increase of renal elasticity was observed after ligation of the renal vein.

• Urinary obstruction is known to increase intrarenal pressure, mostly when acute and complete. The authors' pig study confirmed that elasticity values were highly influenced by the degree of urinary obstruction in a linear fashion (**Fig. 10**). Consequently, urinary obstruction will have to be ruled out before attributing an increased elasticity to tissue changes. Particular attention must be paid to the degree of bladder filling in kidney transplant patients because, due to the shortness of the ureter and to its denervation, a filled bladder may induce a dilatation of the pyelocaliceal system.

NORMAL VALUES AND REPRODUCIBILITY

Only one study reported normal elasticity values within native renal cortex in127 healthy volunteers, ranging in age between 17 and 63 years old.[23] Normal cortical elasticity values were 5.2 ± 2.9 (1–13) kPa and 4.9 ± 2.9 (1–26) kPa in men and

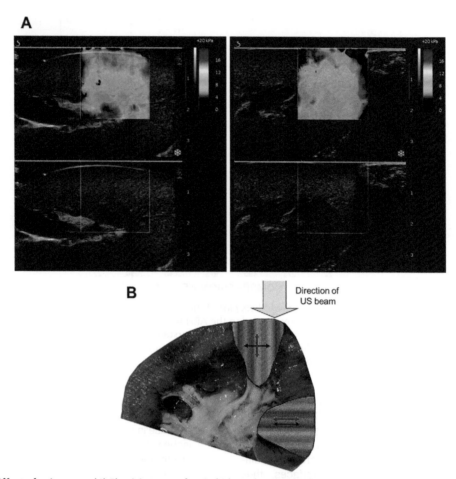

Fig. 8. Effect of anisotropy. (*A*) Elasticity map of a pig kidney showing higher values in the lower pole than on the anterior aspect. (*B*) Macroscopic image of a lower half of a pig kidney showing the corticomedullary differentiation and, superimposed, schematic representation of 2 renal segments: one shows a predominant vertical anisotropy in the direction of US beam, the other a horizontal anisotropy perpendicular to the direction of US beam (*red arrows* illustrate the direction of anisotropy). Axis of propagation of the shear wave (*black arrows*) is perpendicular to the oriented renal structures in the first case and parallel in the second. (*Modified from* Gennisson JL, Grenier N, Combe C, et al. Supersonic shear wave elastography of in vivo pig kidney: influence of blood pressure, urinary pressure and tissue anisotropy. Ultrasound Med Biol 2012;38:1561; with permission.)

women, respectively. The distribution of these values was very large. This dispersion could be due either to a lack of reproducibility of the method, but no information was given related to the number of samplings performed for each patient, or to the difficulties acquiring reproductive elasticity values on native kidney due to their depth. Acquiring stable and reproducible values in renal transplants is much easier than on native kidneys because they are more superficially located, but normally functioning renal transplants cannot be considered as fully normal kidneys and as references.

Ozkan and colleagues[24] measured the interobserver variability in 42 adult renal transplant recipients, using the quasi-static sonoelastography with the calculation of a strain ratio of the central echo complex to the renal parenchyma. For each of the investigators, the elasticity measurements showed large variation. The mean coefficient of variation (CV) of observer 1 and observer 2 was 17% (range: 6%–46%) and 21% (range: 7%–46%), respectively. Interobserver agreement, expressed as intraclass correlation coefficient, was 0.46 (95% CI: 0.05–0.70).

Intraobserver variability was evaluated, with transient elastography, in 12 patients with stable allograft function by Sommerer and colleagues.[18] Stiffness values of both measurements correlated significantly (pole: $r = 0.82$, $P<.0001$; pars

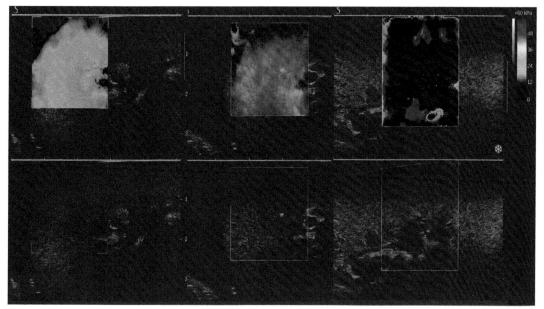

Fig. 9. Effect of perfusion pressure. Example of pig kidney sampled with SSI in normal conditions (mean elasticity 25.6 kPa), after ligation of renal artery (mean elasticity 13.5 kPa) and after ligation of renal vein (mean elasticity 128 kPa).

media: $r = 0.71$, $P = .002$) and varied by 3 ± 14 kPa between the first and second session. Interobserver variability was studied in 10 patients. Stiffness values of both measurements also correlated significantly (pole: $r = 0.78$, $P = .01$; pars media: $r = 0.67$, $P = .03$). Pole and pars media stiffness differed with 6 ± 11 kPa and 1 ± 14 kPa between the measurements of the 2 observers.

Using ARFI, the mean intraobserver CV was 22% for observer 1% and 24% for observer 2.[25] Interobserver agreement, expressed as intraclass correlation coefficient, was 0.31 (95% CI: -0.03–0.60).

Using SSI, intra-observer and interobserver variation coefficients of cortical elasticity were 20% and 12%, respectively.[26] CV range was 10% to 43% for observer 1 and 10% to 35% for observer 2. It is true that CV values could be larger than 30% in some cases, which is not acceptable. However, according to the distribution these CV in this cohort of transplanted patients, a CV <27% was obtained for each observer in 75% of cases.

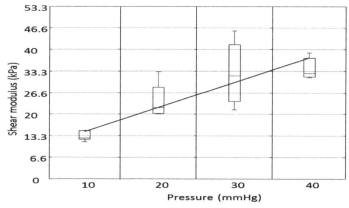

Fig. 10. Effect of urinary pressure. Progressive increase of intrarenal elasticity values with increase of urinary pressure. (*From* Gennisson JL, Grenier N, Combe C, et al. Supersonic shear wave elastography of in vivo pig kidney: influence of blood pressure, urinary pressure and tissue anisotropy. Ultrasound Med Biol 2012;38:1564; with permission.)

These results confirm the low reproducibility of all these techniques requiring several samplings for each measurement.

MEASUREMENT OF RENAL FIBROSIS

An increase in the extracellular matrix synthesis, with excessive fibrillary collagens, characterizes the development of chronic lesions in the glomerular, interstitial, and vascular compartments, leading progressively to end-stage renal failure.[4] Mechanisms participating in these processes are increasingly identified and various therapeutic interventions have been shown to prevent or to favor regression of fibrosis in several experimental models.[5,27] Therefore, development of new noninvasive methods for identification and quantification of fibrosis would be worthwhile.

Preclinical Studies

To the authors' knowledge, only one study attempted to evaluate US elastography in an experimental model[28]: it was a rat model of glomerulosclerosis

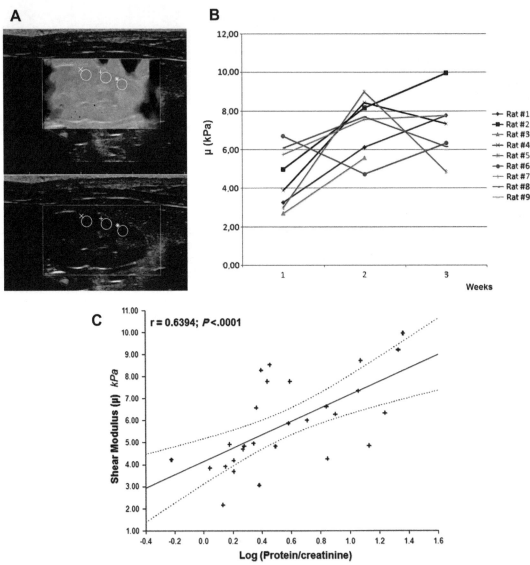

Fig. 11. Preclinical evaluation of renal SSI in a rat model of glomerulosclerosis induced by L-NAME administration. (A) Example of rat kidney sampled with an 8-MHz probe. (B) Progressive increase of intrarenal elasticity values with the development of intrarenal disease. (C) Correlation between renal elasticity values and proteinuria. (Modified from Derieppe M, Delmas Y, Gennisson JL, et al. Detection of intrarenal microstructural changes with supersonic shear wave elastography in rats. Eur Radiol 2012;22:243–50; with permission.)

induced by L-NAME administration, and the objective was use SSI to detect kidney cortex elasticity changes and predicting histopathologic development of fibrosis. Three groups were studied transversally: a control group, a group after 4 weeks of L-NAME administration, and a group after 6 weeks. A fourth group was studied longitudinally before, after 4 weeks, and after 7 weeks of L-NAME administration. This study showed that cortical elasticity values, measured by US SSI, increase with the development of intrarenal disease (**Fig. 11**). When followed longitudinally, these values increased to approximately 76% of their baseline values 4 weeks after the onset of the model and remained stable 3 weeks later. A high degree of correlation between the enhanced renal stiffness and the degree of renal dysfunction, measured by the proteinuria/creatininuria ratio, was very encouraging, but no correlation could be found between the semi-quantitative scoring system (which is the addition of several graded items evaluated qualitatively) and SSI (which is a quantitative value changing linearly).

Study of more fibrotic models is now mandatory to evaluate how elasticity values increase according to the degree of fibrotic tissue deposit. Unfortunately, such models with advanced fibrosis are difficult to obtain in rats. For example, ureteral obstruction is a classical highly fibrotic model but it has the disadvantage of associating fibrosis with a high level of cellularity and with a decrease in the tubular flow and water retention. Therefore, it could not be applied easily to elastographic investigation because increased cellularity and increased intratubular and interstitial hydrostatic pressure, as shown above, would change and bias the elasticity values obtained within the renal parenchyma.

Evaluation of Fibrosis in Native Kidneys

To the authors' knowledge, there is no study of US elastography measurements on native kidneys, probably because of the difficulty in acquiring reproducible values due to their depth (see above).

Evaluation of Renal Transplants

The natural history of IF/TA in transplanted kidneys has been well studied through protocol biopsies. The early phase, which generally occurs during the first years posttransplantation, is characterized by fibrogenesis and the emergence of tubulointerstitial damage due to immunologic phenomena; the late phase is characterized by the worsening of parenchymal lesions (irreversible IF, TA, arteriolar hyalinosis) and the occurrence of glomerular sclerosis leading to graft lost.[7,8] Noninvasive markers of these pathologic changes are lacking and protocol biopsies are still the only reliable tool for the diagnosis of IF/TA.

Several studies have been performed on renal transplants because they are more superficially located, allowing more accurate measurements. Most of them were performed with low-frequency probes (**Fig. 12A**) but high-frequency probes can

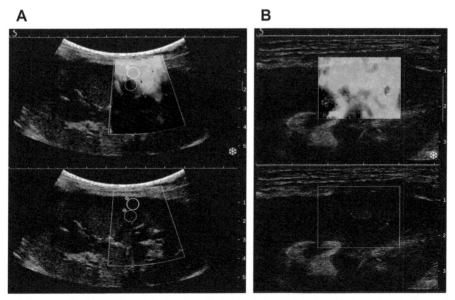

A

B

Fig. 12. Elasticity map of a kidney transplant, using the SSI technique, showing higher values in the cortex than in the medulla, and acquired with a 3- to 5-MHz curved array probe (*A*) and an 8-MHz linear probe (*B*).

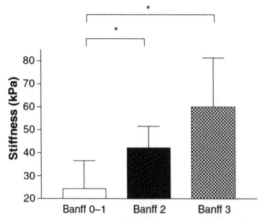

Fig. 13. Parenchymal stiffness measured with Fibroscan in renal transplants with different Banff grades showing a significant difference between patients with Banff grades 0 to 1 versus (*) grade 2 (P: .008), and grade 0 to 1 versus grade 3 (P: .046). (*From Arndt R, Schmidt S, Loddenkemper C, et al. Noninvasive evaluation of renal allograft fibrosis by transient elastography—a pilot study. Transpl Int 2010;23:875; with permission.)*

also be used in very superficial kidneys (see **Fig. 12B**). The correlation between renal elasticity quantification and intrarenal pathologic changes is quite controversial in the literature but the number of enrolled patients for biopsy is quite limited.

Arndt and colleagues,[17] using the Fibroscan, found a correlation between renal stiffness and the degree of IF in a group of 20 patients (**Fig. 13**). A second study with transient elastography was reported by Sommerer and colleagues,[18]

performed on large cohort of 164 transplanted patients. Significantly higher renal stiffness was detected in renal allografts with histologically confirmed advanced fibrosis. The sensitivity and specificity to detect renal allograft fibrosis by transient elastography with a cutoff of 40 kPa were 54% and 73%, respectively.

Using ARFI-SWS, Stock and colleagues[29] found, on 8 patients only, that mean ARFI values showed an average increase of shear-wave velocities of more than 15% in transplants with histologically proven acute rejection, whereas no increase was seen in transplants with other pathologic conditions. Syversveen and colleagues,[25] in 30 patients scheduled for biopsy, did not find any correlation between shear-wave velocities values and the grade of fibrosis. The median values was 2.8 m/s (range: 1.6–3.6), 2.6 m/s (range: 1.8–3.5), and 2.5 m/s (range: 1.6–3) for grade 0 (n = 12), 1 (n = 10), and grades 2/3 (n = 8) fibrosis, respectively. These values did not differ significantly in transplants without and with fibrosis (grade 0 vs grade 1, P = .53 and grade 0 vs grades 2/3, P = .11).

Using SSI, the authors evaluated 49 consecutive kidney transplant recipients scheduled for renal biopsy.[26] None of each individual score of the semi-quantitative Banff classification, including IF (ci), was correlated with the measurement of cortical stiffness. Moreover, cortical stiffness was correlated with neither the level of IF measured by quantitative image analysis nor the scoring and grading of IF/TA (ci + ct). However, renal cortical stiffness did correlate with the sum of the scores of chronic lesions (ci + ct +

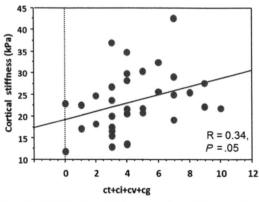
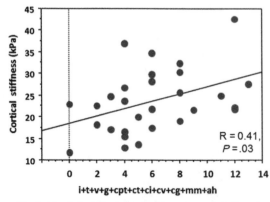

Fig. 14. Relationships between cortical stiffness and sum of individual chronic changes (e) and sum of all pathologic changes (f). Interstitial inflammation (i), tubulitis (t), glomerulitis (g), intimal arteritis (v), peritubular capillaritis (cpt), interstitial fibrosis (ci), tubular atrophy (ct), allograft glomerulopathy (cg), mesangial matrix increase (mm), fibrous intimal thickening (cv), arteriolar hyaline thickening (ah). (*From Grenier N, Poulain S, Lepreux S, et al. Quantitative elastography of renal transplants using supersonic shear imaging: a pilot study. Eur Radiol 2012;22:2144; with permission.)*

cg + cv) and the sum of the scores of all individual lesions (i + t + g + v + cpt + ci + ct + cg + mm + cv + ah) (r = 0.34, P = .05 and r = 0.41, P = .03, respectively).

One possible explanation for such discrepancies is the nonspecificity of stiffness changes related to IF. These results suggest that the degree of renal cortical stiffness does not reflect any specific intrarenal change, such as fibrosis, but rather the association of several renal microlesions, especially chronic lesions (**Fig. 14**).

Renal Tumors

Only one study, to the authors' knowledge, reported shear-wave velocity values in a small series of 12 solid renal cell carcinomas, using ARFI.[30] The values were between 1.61 m/s and 3.97 m/s without any possibility of separating the different tumor types. One example of renal tumor is shown in **Fig. 15**, using the SSI technique. More experience is necessary to evaluate the potential role of elastography in separating benign and malignant tumors.

In summary, quantification of tissue stiffness using US is more complex within the kidney than within the liver. Due to compartmentalization and high tissue heterogeneities, US-guided techniques seem more appropriate. Variability of measurements is increased by the risks of applied transducer pressure on the abdominal wall and to tissue anisotropy. Therefore, more experience is needed in preclinical models and in patient cohorts with pathologic correlation to understand better which are the physical factors of variation and the histopathologic causes of elasticity changes. Noninvasive imaging could participate in this challenge in the near future using functional, structural, or molecular approaches.

REFERENCES

1. Bavu E, Gennisson JL, Couade M, et al. Non-invasive in vivo liver fibrosis staging using supersonic shear imaging: a clinical study. Ultrasound Med Biol 2011;37:1365–73.
2. Castera L, Forns X, Alberti A. Non-invasive evaluation of liver fibrosis using transient elastography. J Hepatol 2008;48:835–47.
3. Palmeri ML, Wang MH, Rouze NC, et al. Noninvasive evaluation of hepatic fibrosis using acoustic radiation force-based shear stiffness in patients with nonalcoholic fatty liver disease. J Hepatol 2011;55:666–72.
4. El Nahas M. The global challenge of chronic kidney disease. Kidney Int 2005;68:2918–29.
5. Chatziantoniou C, Boffa JJ, Tharaux PL, et al. Progression and regression in renal vascular and glomerular fibrosis. Int J Exp Pathol 2004;85:1–11.
6. Ricardo SD, van Goor H, Eddy AA. Macrophage diversity in renal injury and repair. J Clin Invest 2008;118:3522–30.
7. Nankivell BJ, Borrows RJ, Fung CL, et al. The natural history of chronic allograft nephropathy. N Engl J Med 2003;349:2326–33.
8. Stegall MD, Park WD, Larson TS, et al. The histology of solitary renal allografts at 1 and 5 years after transplantation. Am J Transplant 2011;11:698–707.
9. Togao O, Doi S, Kuro-o M, et al. Assessment of renal fibrosis with diffusion-weighted MR imaging: study with murine model of unilateral ureteral obstruction. Radiology 2010;255:772–80.
10. Ophir J, Cespedes I, Ponnekanti H, et al. Elastography: a quantitative method for imaging the elasticity of biological tissues. Ultrason Imaging 1991;13:111–34.
11. Sandrin L, Fourquet B, Hasquenoph JM, et al. Transient elastography: a new noninvasive method for assessment of hepatic fibrosis. Ultrasound Med Biol 2003;29:1705–13.
12. Sandrin L, Tanter M, Gennisson JL, et al. Shear elasticity probe for soft tissues with 1-D transient elastography. IEEE Trans Ultrason Ferroelectr Freq Control 2002;49:436–46.
13. Palmeri ML, Wang MH, Dahl JJ, et al. Quantifying hepatic shear modulus in vivo using acoustic radiation force. Ultrasound Med Biol 2008;34:546–58.
14. Bercoff J, Tanter M, Fink M. Supersonic shear imaging: a new technique for soft tissue elasticity mapping. IEEE Trans Ultrason Ferroelectr Freq Control 2004;51:396–409.

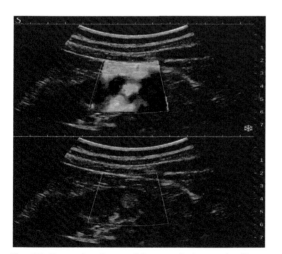

Fig. 15. Example of a small hyperechoic renal cell carcinoma evaluated with SSI technique: tumor elasticity ratio between tumor and renal parenchyma was 2.9.

15. Emelianov SY, Lubinski MA, Weitzel WF, et al. Elasticity imaging for early detection of renal pathology. Ultrasound Med Biol 1995;21:871–83.
16. Weitzel WF, Kim K, Rubin JM, et al. Feasibility of applying ultrasound strain imaging to detect renal transplant chronic allograft nephropathy. Kidney Int 2004;65:733–6.
17. Arndt R, Schmidt S, Loddenkemper C, et al. Noninvasive evaluation of renal allograft fibrosis by transient elastography–a pilot study. Transpl Int 2010; 23:871–7.
18. Sommerer C, Scharf M, Seitz C, et al. Assessment of renal allograft fibrosis by transient elastography. Transpl Int 2013;26(5):545–51.
19. Syversveen T, Midtvedt K, Berstad AE, et al. Tissue elasticity estimated by acoustic radiation force impulse quantification depends on the applied transducer force: an experimental study in kidney transplant patients. Eur Radiol 2012;22:2130–7.
20. Ries M, Jones RA, Basseau F, et al. Diffusion tensor MRI of the human kidney. J Magn Reson Imaging 2001;14:42–9.
21. Gennisson JL, Grenier N, Combe C, et al. Supersonic shear wave elastography of in vivo pig kidney: influence of blood pressure, urinary pressure and tissue anisotropy. Ultrasound Med Biol 2012;38: 1559–67.
22. Warner L, Yin M, Glaser KJ, et al. Noninvasive in vivo assessment of renal tissue elasticity during graded renal ischemia using MR elastography. Invest Radiol 2011;46:509–14.
23. Arda K, Ciledag N, Aktas E, et al. Quantitative assessment of normal soft-tissue elasticity using shear-wave ultrasound elastography. AJR Am J Roentgenol 2011;197:532–6.
24. Ozkan F, Yavuz YC, Inci MF, et al. Interobserver variability of ultrasound elastography in transplant kidneys: correlations with clinical-Doppler parameters. Ultrasound Med Biol 2013;39:4–9.
25. Syversveen T, Brabrand K, Midtvedt K, et al. Assessment of renal allograft fibrosis by acoustic radiation force impulse quantification–a pilot study. Transpl Int 2011;24:100–5.
26. Grenier N, Poulain S, Lepreux S, et al. Quantitative elastography of renal transplants using supersonic shear imaging: a pilot study. Eur Radiol 2012;22: 2138–46.
27. Boffa JJ, Lu Y, Placier S, et al. Regression of renal vascular and glomerular fibrosis: role of angiotensin II receptor antagonism and matrix metalloproteinases. J Am Soc Nephrol 2003;14: 1132–44.
28. Derieppe M, Delmas Y, Gennisson JL, et al. Detection of intrarenal microstructural changes with supersonic shear wave elastography in rats. Eur Radiol 2012;22:243–50.
29. Stock KF, Klein BS, Cong MT, et al. ARFI-based tissue elasticity quantification and kidney graft dysfunction: first clinical experiences. Clin Hemorheol Microcirc 2011;49:527–35.
30. Clevert DA, Stock K, Klein B, et al. Evaluation of Acoustic Radiation Force Impulse (ARFI) imaging and contrast-enhanced ultrasound in renal tumors of unknown etiology in comparison to histological findings. Clin Hemorheol Microcirc 2009; 43:95–107.

Ultrasound Evaluation of Renal Masses: Gray-scale, Doppler, and More

Seung H. Kim, MD[a],*, Jeong Y. Cho, MD[a],
Sang Y. Kim, MD[a], Kyung C. Moon, MD[b],
Cheol Kwak, MD[c], Hyeon H. Kim, MD[c]

KEYWORDS

• Renal mass • Renal cell carcinoma • Imaging • Ultrasonography

KEY POINTS

- Gray-scale ultrasound (US) alone is not enough for renal mass evaluation.
- Doppler US has added value in differentiation between
  - True mass versus pseudomass
  - Cystic versus solid mass
  - Benign versus malignant renal tumors
  - Typical clear cell renal cell carcinomas (RCCs) versus other type RCCs
  - Hyperechoic RCCs versus angiomyolipomas
- Doppler US is also useful in detection of RCC in end-stage renal disease.
- Contrast-enhanced US may be a problem-solving technique for indeterminate renal masses.

INTRODUCTION

Ultrasound (US) is commonly the first step in the imaging evaluation of renal masses, where its main role is detection and characterization. Usually computed tomography (CT) or magnetic resonance imaging (MRI) is needed for further characterization if a renal mass appears to have solid parts. Infrequently, US may provide information on renal masses that was equivocal at CT or MRI.[1]

Increased detection of renal cell carcinomas (RCCs) probably results from increased use of US in the general population, technical advances of imaging studies that could depict smaller masses, and possibly a real increase of incidence of RCCs.[2] This results in increased detection of benign renal neoplasms and non-neoplastic masses also, so the differentiation between neoplastic and non-neoplastic lesions and between benign and malignant neoplasms has become more important.[3] US has difficulty in detecting small renal masses that have isoechogenicity with renal parenchyma, especially when the mass is totally intraparenchymal or at a polar region (**Fig. 1**).

US has many advantages over other imaging modalities, especially in that it is easy and quick to perform. In a study comparing the size of renal mass measured at various imaging modalities, US did not appear to be inferior to CT or MRI, and so US might be useful for long-term active surveillance of a renal mass with less cost and radiation exposure.[4,5]

US is not an adequate imaging modality for assessment of local extent of the renal tumor

[a] Department of Radiology, Institute of Radiation Medicine, Clinical Research Institute, Seoul National University College of Medicine, Seoul National University Hospital, 101 Daehak-ro, Jongno-gu, 110-744 Seoul, Korea; [b] Department of Pathology, Clinical Research Institute, Seoul National University College of Medicine, Seoul National University Hospital, 101 Daehak-ro, Jongno-gu, 110-744 Seoul, Korea; [c] Department of Urology, Clinical Research Institute, Seoul National University College of Medicine, Seoul National University Hospital, 101 Daehak-ro, Jongno-gu, 110-744 Seoul, Korea
* Corresponding author.
E-mail address: kimshrad@snu.ac.kr

Ultrasound Clin 8 (2013) 565–579
http://dx.doi.org/10.1016/j.cult.2013.07.002

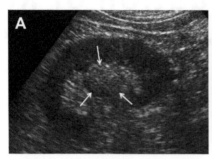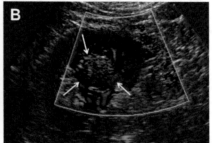

Fig. 1. A 52-year-old man with papRCC. (*A*) US in longitudinal plane shows a 3 cm-sized renal mass in the central part of the left kidney with homogeneous echogenicity (*arrows*) that is almost identical to that of renal parenchyma. (*B*) PDUS shows that the mass (*arrows*) is hypovascular.

and regional lymph node metastasis. However, the extent of tumor thrombus is usually well demonstrated with US (**Fig. 2**). Evaluation of sliding between renal tumor and adjacent organs such as the liver or spleen provides information on direct invasion of those organs by the renal tumor.[6] US is useful for guiding biopsy or minimally invasive ablative therapies for renal mass. Intraoperative US is useful in localizing small intraparechymal tumors or monitoring extraction of tumor thrombus during surgery.

Although it is well known that US is accurate in differentiating between cystic and solid renal masses, it is also known that often this differentiation is difficult. One can make a diagnosis of simple renal cyst if a renal mass is round, well-demarcated, anechoic, and accompanies posterior acoustic enhancement. If a renal mass does not have any of these findings, that renal mass is not likely a simple renal cyst, and it should be evaluated further. Sometimes a homogeneous solid renal mass may be difficult to differentiate from a simple renal cyst if it accompanies sonic enhancement and edge shadowing (**Fig. 3**).

There have been continuous technical advances in US in the area of gray-scale US, including tissue harmonic imaging. There also have been improvements in Doppler US, including color Doppler US (CDUS), power Doppler US (PDUS), and spectral Doppler US (SDUS). Elastography and contrast-enhanced US (CEUS) can be used in the evaluation of renal masses.

RENAL MASS DETECTION

With wide use of abdominal US, RCCs are being detected more. US detection of renal mass is based on gray-scale and Doppler US findings. Harmonic imaging may improve contrast resolution and cause less artifact.[7]

The first step to detecting and characterizing a renal mass is to distinguish it from a pseudomass, most common of which is a prominent column of Bertin. Gray-scale US may not be enough to differentiate between a true renal mass and a prominent column. CDUS or PDUS may be useful in this differentiation. Basically, dominant vessels are displaced around the lesion in a true renal mass, while vessels run through the lesion in a pseudomass (**Figs. 4** and **5**).

RENAL MASS CHARACTERIZATION

If a solid renal mass is found in an adult, the differential diagnosis is basically between an RCC and

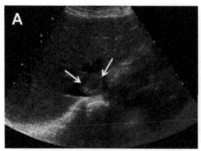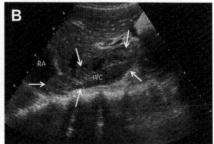

Fig. 2. A 70-year-old woman with RCC with thrombus in the renal vein and inferior vena cava. US of the inferior vena cava (IVC) in transverse (*A*) and longitudinal (*B*) planes shows a large thrombus (*arrows*) in the IVC. Note that the longitudinal US well demonstrates the cranial end of the thrombus bulging into the right atrium (RA).

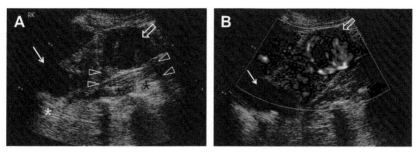

Fig. 3. A 62-year-old man with RCC and simple renal cyst in the same kidney. (A) Longitudinal US of the right kidney shows 2 renal masses. A mass in the cranial part (*arrow*) has findings of typical renal cyst (ie, round shape, well-defined margin, imperceptible wall, anechoic, and posterior sonic enhancement) (*white asterisk*). The other mass (*open arrow*) also appears round, well-demarcated, and accompanies subtle posterior acoustic enhancement (*black asterisks*), but it has homogeneous medium-level echo. Also note that the mass has edge shadowing (*arrowheads*) along the margin of the mass. (B) Longitudinal PDUS shows that the mass in the cranial part (*arrow*) is avascular, and the mass in the caudal part (*open arrow*) is very hypervascular.

other renal tumors, including benign renal lesions such as angiomyolipomas (AMLs), adenoma and oncocytoma, and other malignancies such as lymphoma, renal sarcoma, and metastasis.

Renal masses other than a simple cyst and a solid RCC may be collectively called indeterminate renal masses. They can be categorized according to their internal structure into: mainly

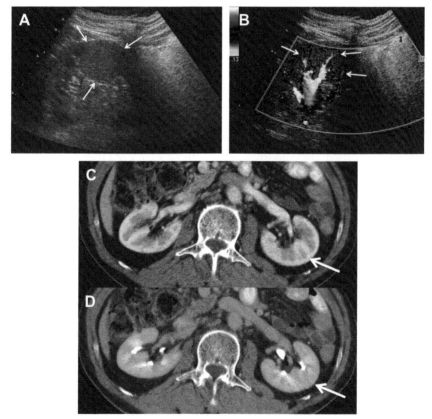

Fig. 4. A 66-year old man with pseudomass due to prominent column of Bertin. (A) US of the left kidney in the transverse plane shows a mass-like lesion that has homogeneous medium-level echo (*arrows*). (B) CDUS of the mass shows vessels (*arrows*) that traverse through the mass. Contrast-enhanced CT of the kidney in the cortical phase (C) and delayed excretory phase (D) shows no evidence of the mass. The area of the renal parenchyma that appeared as a mass-like lesion at US (*arrow*) shows contrast enhancement same as the normal renal cortex.

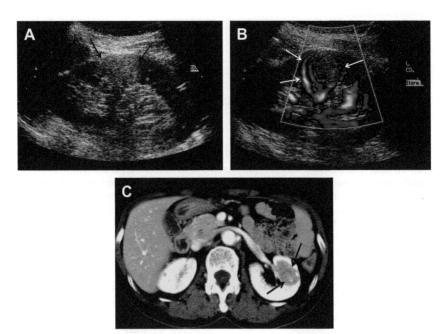

Fig. 5. A 55-year-old woman with cpRCC. (*A*) US of the left kidney in the longitudinal plane shows a mass-like lesion that has homogeneous high-level echo (*arrows*). This US finding is very similar to that of **Fig. 4**A. (*B*) PDUS of the mass shows vessels (*arrows*) displaced by the mass. This finding is different from that of **Fig. 4**B. (*C*) Contrast-enhanced CT shows heterogeneously enhancing mass (*arrows*) in the left kidney.

cystic, mixed cystic and solid, and mainly solid renal masses, with increasing degree of suspicion of malignancy.

Characterization of Cystic Renal Masses

The simple cyst is the most common renal mass encountered. Well-established characteristics of a simple renal cyst include sharp borders, an imperceptible wall, anechoic contents, and strong posterior sonic enhancement. Varying degrees of cyst complexity are often shown at US such as low-level internal echoes, septa, thick walls, calcification, and mural nodularity.

In 1986, Bosniak proposed a 4-category classification system in evaluating cystic renal masses.[8] He proposed this classification with CT findings, but it can be applied to US findings also. A class 1 lesion indicates a clearly simple cyst; a class 2 lesion indicates a minimally complicated cyst with thin septa, most likely a benign cyst, and a class 3 lesion is a more complicated lesion that has complex and thick septa, often solid nodules. Because a class 3 lesion has a high possibility of malignancy, further evaluation or surgery is necessary. A class 4 lesion is obviously a malignant lesion, and the patient definitely needs surgery. With this classification system, always the problem was differentiation between class 2 and 3, so in 1993, Bosniak added class class 2F, which is

a little bit more complicated than class 2, but less than class 3, and so needs close follow-up.[9]

About 15% of RCCs are radiologically cystic. The wall and septa of the cystic RCC are usually thick and irregular, and often there are solid nodules along the inner wall or septa (**Fig. 6**). Multilocular cystic RCC is a rare low-grade malignancy with an excellent prognosis. It has a multilocular cystic appearance with irregular thick septa, but it usually does not show a discrete nodular lesion (**Fig. 7**).[10]

CDUS or PDUS can be helpful in evaluating indeterminate cystic renal masses by depicting vascularity in the mass. On the contrary, absence of flow signals suggests high likelihood of benign lesion, either neoplastic or non-neoplastic (**Fig. 8**). However, presence of flow signals in the septa does not always indicate malignancy. Benign neoplasms such as multilocular cystic nephroma or renal hemangioma may show multilocular cystic appearance with flow signals in the septa. Flow signals on CDUS or PDUS should be confirmed by using spectral Doppler US (**Fig. 9**), because artifacts such as twinkling artifact may mimic flow signals (**Fig. 10**).[11]

Characterization of Solid Renal Masses

As RCC is the most common solid renal neoplasm, diagnosis of a renal mass is virtually

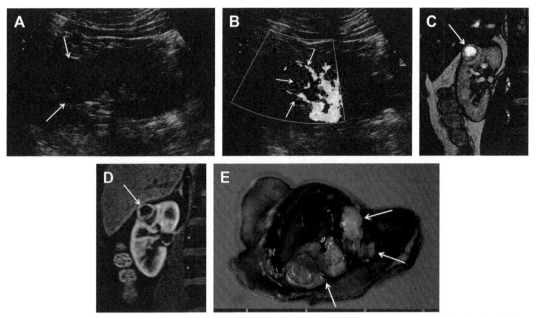

Fig. 6. Cystic RCC of clear cell type in a 65-year-old man. (A) US of the right kidney in the longitudinal plane shows a mass of mixed cystic and solid portions (*arrows*) in the upper pole. (B) The mass has vascularity in the peripheral solid parts (*arrows*). (C) T2-weighted MR image in the coronal plane shows a thick-walled cystic mass (*arrow*) in the upper pole of the right kidney. (D) Contrast-enhanced T1-weighted MR image shows strong enhancement of the thick peripheral wall (*arrow*). (E) Partial nephrectomy was done, and the cut surface of the resected specimen shows a cystic mass with peripheral nodular neoplastic lesions (*arrows*).

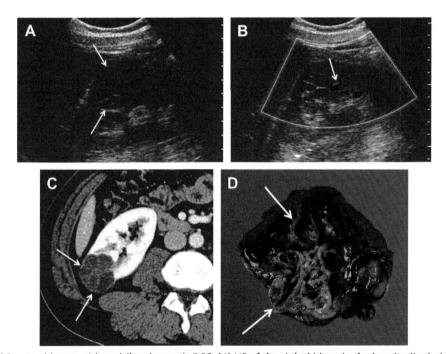

Fig. 7. A 36-year-old man with multilocular cystic RCC. (A) US of the right kidney in the longitudinal plane shows a cystic mass (*arrows*) with multiple fine septa. (B) PDUS of the mass shows focal flow signal (*arrow*) in the septa. (C) Contrast-enhanced CT shows a cystic mass (*arrows*) with subtle enhancement of the septa. (D) Cut surface of the resected specimen shows multiple septa in the mass (*arrows*) without definite nodular lesions.

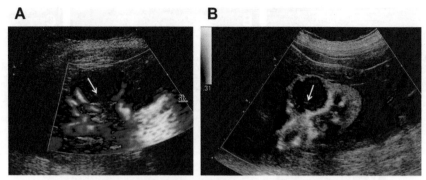

Fig. 8. A 64-year-old woman with benign septated renal cyst. (*A*) PDUS of the right kidney shows a cystic mass with a thin septum (*arrow*) that does not show flow signal. (*B*) CEUS shows no evidence of enhancement of the septum (*arrow*).

a differentiation of RCC from other neoplasms. A solid mass in the adult kidney can be considered an RCC unless there is strong evidence that suggests other diagnosis. AMLs frequently show characteristic US findings, but oncocytomas usually do not. Lymphomas, metastases, and various sarcomas comprise other part of solid renal tumors. As lymphomas and metastases have unique clinical settings, most cases can be diagnosed easily (**Fig. 11**). Sarcomas are unusually large and have a grotesque appearance.

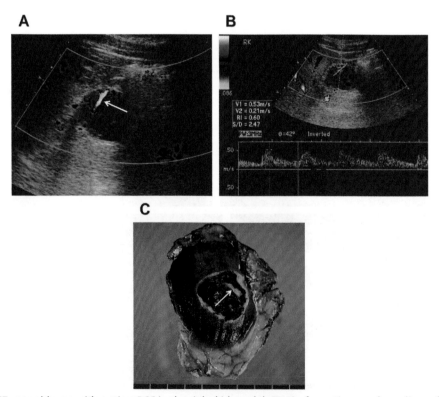

Fig. 9. A 57-year-old man with cystic ccRCC in the right kidney. (*A*) CDUS of a cystic mass shows linear flow signal in a septa (*arrow*). (*B*) SDUS performed at the septa shows clear arterial flow signal. (*C*) Nephrectomy was done, and the cut surface of the mass shows an internal septum (*arrow*) corresponding to the one that showed flow signals on Doppler US.

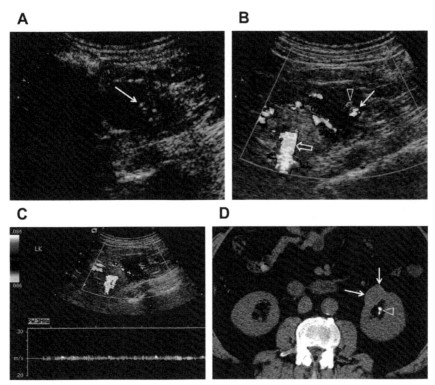

Fig. 10. A 60-year-old man with a benign cyst with echogenic content and a peripheral nodular lesion with twinkling artifact. This artifact may be confused with true flow signal. (*A*) US of the left kidney shows a cystic mass with echogenic nodular lesion in the peripheral portion (*arrow*). (*B*) CDUS of the mass shows a twinkling color artifact (*arrow*) located not in the echogenic nodular lesion itself (*arrowhead*) but posterior to it. Also note strong twinkling artifact in the hilar portion of the kidney due to a calyceal stone (*open arrow*). (*C*) SDUS performed at the twinkling artifact in the cystic mass shows bidirectional artifactual signals. (*D*) Nonenhanced CT scan shows a high attenuation cyst (*arrows*) and calyceal stones (*arrowhead*) in the left kidney.

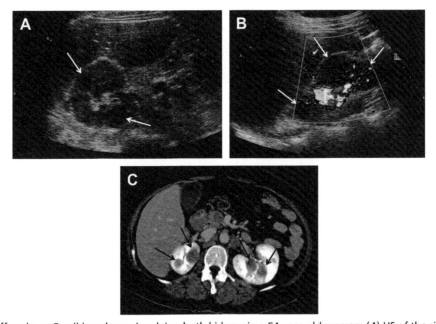

Fig. 11. Diffuse large B-cell lymphoma involving both kidneys in a 54-year-old woman. (*A*) US of the right kidney in transverse plane shows multiple hypoechoic masses (*arrows*). (*B*) CDUS of the right kidney shows hypovascular nature of the masses (*arrows*). (*C*) Contrast-enhanced CT shows multiple hypoenhancing nodular masses in both kidneys (*arrows*).

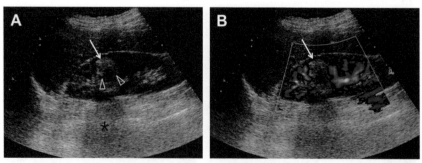

Fig. 12. A 66-year-old woman with AML. (*A*) US of the right kidney in longitudinal plane shows a hyperechoic mass (*arrow*). The echogenicity of the mass is similar to the hilar echogencity. Note that the posterior margin of the mass is poorly demarcated (*arrowheads*), and the mass accompanies posterior sonic attenuation (*asterisk*). (*B*) PDUS shows hypovascularity of the mass (*arrow*).

DIFFERENTIATION BETWEEN RCC AND AML

AML is a nonencapsulated, slow-growing, and expansile mass. It is a hamartoma of the kidney and is composed of a varying proportion of blood vessels, smooth muscle, and fat. Because AML has various components of tissues, its overall echogenicity is hyperechoic and heterogeneous. The echogenicity of AMLs, especially small ones, is similar to or even higher than that of the renal sinus, and it is usually much higher than the

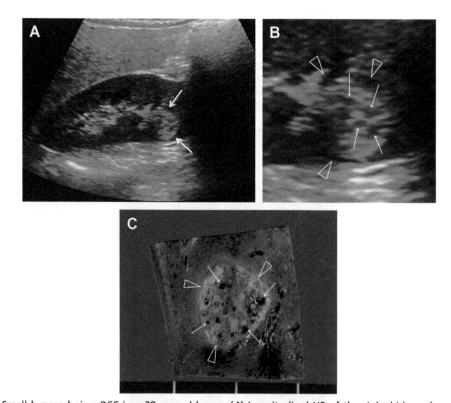

Fig. 13. Small hyperechoic ccRCC in a 28-year-old man. (*A*) Longitudinal US of the right kidney shows a round hyperechoic mass in the lower polar region. The echogenicity of the mass is higher than that of the renal parenchyma but lower than renal hilar echogencity. Note that the renal mass has hypoechoic peripheral halo (*arrows*). (*B*). Magnified image of the mass well demonstrates hypoechoic peritumoral halo (*arrowheads*) and small intratumoral cysts (*arrows*). (*C*) Cut surface of the resected specimen shows a renal mass surrounded by a whitish fibrous pseudocapsule (*arrowheads*) that corresponds to the peritumoral hypoechoic halo on US. Note small intratumoral cysts filled with dark hemorrhage (*arrows*).

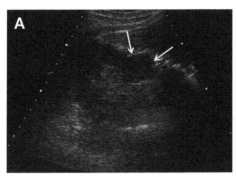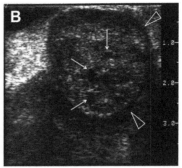

Fig. 14. Small isoechoic ccRCC in a 60-year-old man. (A) US of the right kidney shows a small round mass of iso-echogenicity (arrows). (B) On intraoperative US, the mass shows subtle hyperechogenicity. Also note peritumoral hypoechoic halo (arrowheads) and small intratumoral cysts (arrows).

hyperechogenicity of small RCCs. AMLs usually have posterior sonic attenuation with poorly defined posterior margin (Fig. 12). The diagnosis of AML is straightforward if it has macroscopic fat, which is clearly seen on nonenhanced CT. However, considerable proportions of AMLs are with minimal amounts of fat, which may make it difficult to distinguish them from RCCs.

Approximately one-third of small RCCs (3 cm in diameter or less) show marked hyperechogenicty that may mimic AML.[12] In addition to hyperechogenicity, small RCCs often show intratumoral cysts and a thin hypoechoic rim (Figs. 13 and 14). Other rare renal tumors (eg, renal metastasis from osteogenic sarcoma or thyroid cancer) also may be hyperechoic.[13] As RCCs grow, they usually show heterogeneous hypoechogenicity caused by internal necrosis and hemorrhage.

There have been trials for quantitative comparison of echogenicity or sonic attenuation between AMLs and hyperechoic RCCs.[14–16] In one study, the gray-scale value of the renal sinus was designated as 100% and the renal cortex as 0%, and the relative echogenicity of the renal mass was measured in a percent value. Most of RCCs had the relative gray-scale value less than 80%, while almost all of the AMLs had over 80% value.[14] This way of comparison of relative echogenicity is simple and can be easily measured on a PACS system (Fig. 15).[15] Small AMLs and hyperechoic RCCs show different vascular patterns.[17] At CDUS or PDUS, AMLs usually show no flow or mottled focal intratumoral flow (Fig. 16), while RCCs usually show peripheral displaced vessels (Fig. 17). In differentiating between AML and hyperechoic RCC, confirmation by nonenhanced CT is advised. With CT, detection of macroscopic fat in a renal mass is virtually diagnostic for AML. If no such macroscopic fat is found, further characterization with contrast-enhanced CT or MRI is needed.

RCC, HISTOLOGIC SUBTYPES

There are various histologic subtypes of RCCs, of which clear cell RCC (ccRCC) is the most common, comprising about 70% to 85% of all RCCs. About 10% of RCCs are papillary type RCCs

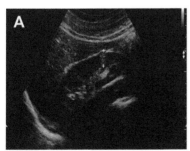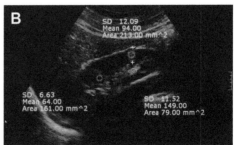

Fig. 15. Small ccRCC in a 48-year-old man. (A) Longitudinal US of the right kidney shows a small hyperechoic mass (between cursors) in the lower polar region. The echogenicity of the mass is higher than that of the renal parenchyma but lower than renal hilar echogencity. (B) Measurement of relative echogenicity on PACS system. In this case, relative echogenicity of the renal mass was 65%, with assignment of 0% to the cortical echogenicity and 100% to the hilar echogenicity.

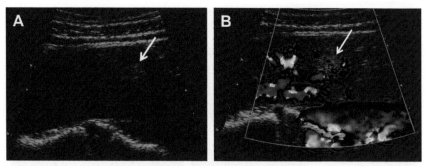

Fig. 16. AML with minimal fat in a 44-year-old woman. (*A*) Longitudinal US of the right kidney shows a small hyperechoic renal mass (*arrow*). (*B*) CDUS of the mass shows mottled intratumoral flow signals (*arrow*). Partial nephrectomy was done, and the mass was confirmed to be AML.

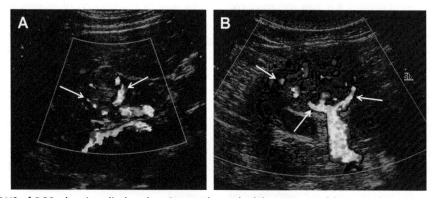

Fig. 17. CDUS of RCCs showing displaced peritumoral vessels. (*A*) A 30-year-old man with cpRCC. CDUS of the right kidney shows a hyperechoic mass with displaced vessels around the mass (*arrows*). (*B*) A 79-year-old man with ccRCC. CDUS of the right kidney shows a hypervascular renal mass with displaced peritumoral vessels (*arrows*).

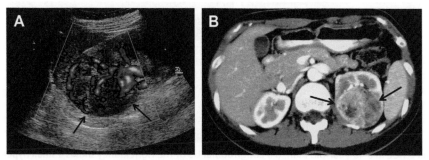

Fig. 18. A 27-year-old woman with ccRCC. (*A*) PDUS of the left kidney shows a hypervascular renal mass (*arrows*). (*B*) Contrast-enhanced CT scan in the cortical phase shows heterogeneous enhancement of the renal mass (*arrows*). Note that the degree of enhancement of the enhancing portion of the mass is as strong as the renal cortical enhancement.

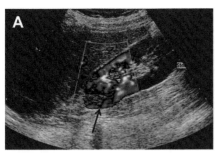
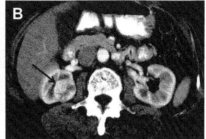

Fig. 19. A 46-year-old woman with small ccRCC. (A) PDUS of the right kidney shows a small hypervascular renal mass (arrows). (B) Contrast-enhanced CT scan in the cortical phase shows strong enhancement of the renal mass (arrow). Note that the mass shows heterogeneous enhancement, and the degree of enhancement of the enhancing portion is as strong as the renal cortical enhancement.

(papRCCs), and about 5% are chromophobe RCCs (cpRCC). Other rare subtypes include collecting duct carcinoma and unclassified type RCC. Sarcomatoid variant, previously known as sarcomatoid type RCC, is not considered as a type of its own, because it arises from all other types of carcinomas.

Familiarity with various imaging findings characteristic of RCCs according to histologic subtypes is important, because there are significant differences in prognosis among different histologic subtypes.[18] There is a tendency of earlier and stronger enhancement in ccRCCs than other subtypes (Fig. 18). At early arterial phase of contrast-enhanced CT, a renal mass that enhances stronger than the renal cortex is characteristic of ccRCC (Fig. 19). This enhancement pattern can be seen at CEUS also (Fig. 20). In contrast, papRCCs often show homogeneous appearance of variable echogenicity on gray-scale US and hypovascularity on Doppler US (Fig. 21). US findings of cpRCCs are in between those of ccRCCs and papRCCs (Fig. 22).

RENAL MASS IN END-STAGE RENAL DISEASE

About one-third of cases with end-stage renal disease (ESRD) are associated with acquired renal

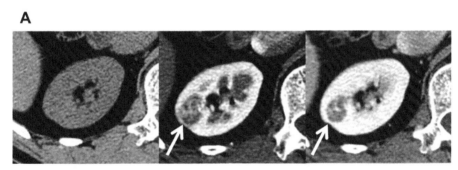

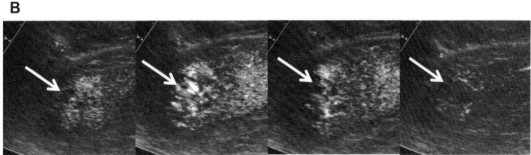

Fig. 20. A 56-year-old man with small ccRCC. (A) Nonenhanced (left) and contrast-enhanced CT scans in the cortical (middle) and nephrographic (right) phases show heterogeneous enhancement of the mass (arrow). (B). Contrast-enhanced US obtained 15, 20, 30, and 40 seconds after injection of contrast agent (from left to right, respectively) shows early enhancement and rapid washout of the mass (arrow).

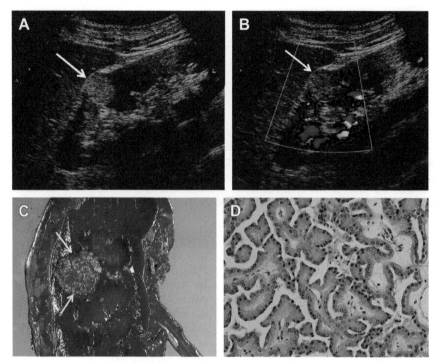

Fig. 21. A 45-year-old man with papRCC. (*A*) Longitudinal US of the right kidney shows a small round renal mass of homogeneous hyperechogenicity (*arrow*). (*B*) CDUS shows the hypovascular nature of the mass (*arrow*). (*C*) Cut surface of the resected specimen shows the fine velvety appearance of the mass (*arrows*). (*D*) Photomicrograph of the mass shows the papillary architecture of the mass.

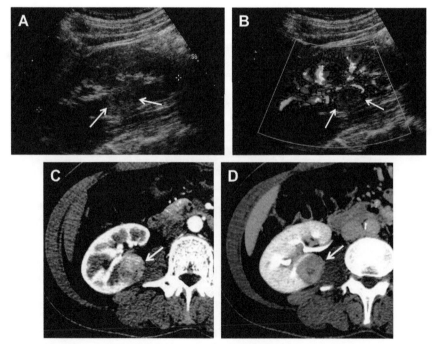

Fig. 22. A 48-year-old woman with cpRCC. (*A*) Longitudinal US of the right kidney shows an ill-demarcated mass of slight hyperechogenicity (*arrows*). (*B*). CDUS of the mass shows slight hypervascularity of the mass (*arrows*). Contrast-enhanced CT scans in the cortical (*C*) and excretory (*D*) phases show enhancement of the mass (*arrow*), not as strong as that of ccRCC.

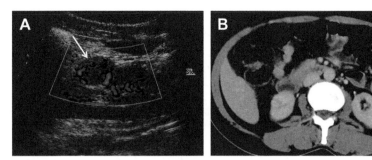

Fig. 23. Pseudotumor of the kidney in a 40-year-old woman with ESRD. (*A*) Longitudinal PDUS of the left kidney shows a mass-like lesion (*arrow*) of isoechogenicity and isovascularity. (*B*) Contrast-enhanced CT scan in the excretory phase shows bulging of renal contour in the left kidney due to focal hypertrophy (*arrow*). Note that the enhancement of the lesion is not different from that in other parts of the kidney.

cystic disease. Patients with ESRD also show an increased incidence of solid renal masses, most common of which is renal pseudotumor. True renal tumors seen in patients with ESRD are RCCs of various histologic subtypes, adenomas, and oncocytomas. Two subtypes of RCC that appear unique to ESRD are acquired cystic disease associated RCC and clear-cell papillary RCC of end-stage kidney disease.[19]

Differentiation of an RCC from a pseudotumor is important in a patient with ESRD. Doppler US is useful in this differentiation. If a renal mass shows similar vascularity at CDUS or PDUS and similar Doppler spectral pattern at SDUS, the mass is likely a pseudotumor (**Fig. 23**). If a renal mass shows hypervascularity and lower resistance compared with the rest of renal parenchyma, the mass is probably an RCC (**Fig. 24**). The reason for this difference of Doppler spectral pattern is the difference between the vascular wall of normal tissue and the malignant tumor (**Fig. 25**). The Doppler spectrum of malignant lesion usually

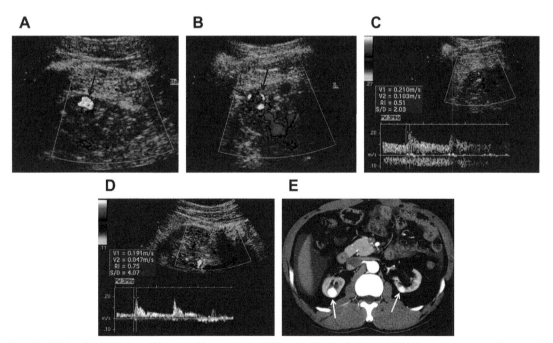

Fig. 24. Bilateral ccRCCs in a 43-year-old man with ESRD. (*A*) CDUS of the right kidney shows a small mass of strong hypervascularity (*arrow*). (*B*) CDUS of the left kidney shows a small mass of slight hypervascularity (*arrows*). (*C*). SDUS obtained in the left renal mass shows low-resistance arterial flow (Resistive Index 0.51). (*D*) SDUS obtained within the renal parenchyma, out of the mass, shows high-resistance arterial flow (Resistive Index 0.75). (*E*). Contrast-enhanced CT scan in the cortical phase shows strong enhancement of the renal masses in both kidneys (*arrow*).

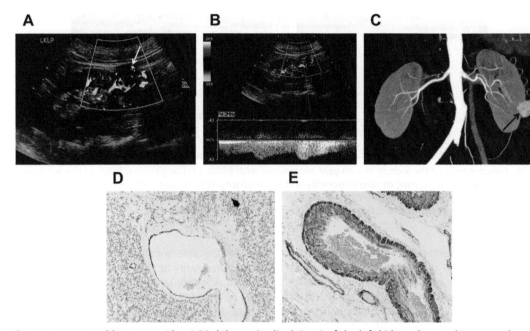

Fig. 25. A 52-year-old woman with ccRCC. (*A*) Longitudinal CDUS of the left kidney shows a hypervascular renal mass in the lower polar region (*arrow*). (*B*). SDUS performed in the renal mass shows a low-resistance arterial flow pattern. (*C*) CT angiography shows an enhancing mass (*arrow*) in the left kidney with prominent feeding vessels. (*D*) Photomicrograph of an arterial structure in the renal mass shows a deficient media layer in the arterial wall. (*E*) Photomicrograph of an arterial structure in the uninvolved renal parenchyma shows a normal arterial wall with distinct media layer.

shows high velocity and low resistance, where high velocity indicates the presence of arteriovenous fistula, and low resistance is due to a deficient media layer in the arterial wall.[20,21]

US-GUIDED RENAL BIOPSY

Small renal masses presumed to be RCC at preoperative imaging studies turn out to be benign at pathology in 13% to 16% of cases, a substantial proportion. The percentage of benign tumors decreased from 46.3% for those less than 1 cm to 6.3% for those 7 cm or greater.[22–24] That is a reason why renal tumor biopsies are increasingly being used. Renal tumor biopsies are used increasingly also in metastatic patients before starting therapy, in follow-up surveillance, and in ablative therapies. The accuracy of renal mass biopsy is being improved, with a decreasing rate of nondiagnostic results.[25] For small renal masses, CT-guided biopsy is being used more frequently.

REFERENCES

1. Helenon O, Correas JM, Balleyguier C, et al. Ultrasound of renal tumors. Eur Radiol 2001;11: 1890–901.

2. Mindrup SR, Pierre JS, Dahmoush L, et al. The prevalence of renal cell carcinoma diagnosed at autopsy. BJU Int 2005;95:31–3.

3. Marhuenda A, Martín MI, Deltoro C, et al. Radiologic evaluation of small renal masses: pretreatment management. Adv Urol 2008. http://dx.doi.org/10.1155/2008/415848.

4. Mucksavage P, Ramchandani P, Malkowicz B, et al. Is ultrasound imaging inferior to computed tomography or magnetic resonance imaging in evaluating renal mass size? Urology 2012;79:28–31.

5. Jewett MA, Mattar K, Basiuk J, et al. Active surveillance of small renal masses: progression patterns of early stage kidney cancer. Eur Urol 2011;60: 39–44.

6. Lim JH, Ko YT, Lee DH. Sonographic sliding sign in localization of right upper quadrant mass. J Ultrasound Med 1990;8:455–9.

7. Heller MT, Tublin ME. Detection and characterization of renal masses by ultrasound: a practical guide. Ultrasound Q 2007;23:269–78.

8. Bosniak MA. The current radiological approach to renal cysts. Radiology 1986;158:1–10.

9. Bosniak MA. Problems in the radiologic diagnosis of renal parenchyma tumors. Urol Clin North Am 1993; 20:217–30.

10. Hindman NM, Bosniak MA, Rosenkrantz AB, et al. Multilocular cystic renal cell carcinoma: comparison

of imaging and pathologic findings. AJR Am J Roentgenol 2012;198:W20–6.

11. Lee JY, Kim SH, Cho JY, et al. Color and power Doppler twinkling artifacts from urinary stones: clinical observations and phantom studies. AJR Am J Roentgenol 2001;176:1441–5.

12. Forman HP, Middleton WD, Melson GL, et al. Hyperechoic renal cell carcinomas at US. Radiology 1993; 188:431–4.

13. Ahmed M, Aslam M, Ahmed J, et al. Renal metastases from thyroid cancer masquerading as renal angiomyolipoma on ultrasonography. J Ultrasound Med 2006;25:1459–64.

14. Sim JS, Seo CS, Kim SH, et al. Differentiation of small hyperechoic renal cell carcinoma from angiomyolipoma: computer-aided tissue echo quantification. J Ultrasound Med 1999;18:261–4.

15. Lee MS, Cho JY, Kim SH. Ultrasonographic differentiation of small angiomyolipoma from renal cell carcinoma by measuring relative echogenicity on PACS. J Korean Soc Ultrasound Med 2010;29:105–13.

16. Taniguchi N, Itoh K, Nakamura S, et al. Differentiation of renal cell carcinomas from angiomyolipomas by ultrasonic frequency dependent attenuation. J Urol 1997;157:1242–5.

17. Jinzaki M, Ohkuma K, Tanimoto A, et al. Small solid renal lesions: usefulness of power Doppler US. Radiology 1998;209:543–50.

18. Prasad SR, Humphrey PA, Catena JR, et al. Common and uncommon histologic subtypes of renal cell carcinoma: imaging spectrum with pathologic correlation. Radiographics 2006;26: 1795–810.

19. Tickoo SK, dePeralta-Venturina MN, Harik LR, et al. Spectrum of epithelial neoplasms in end-stage renal disease: an experience from 66 tumor-bearing kidneys with emphasis on histologic patterns distinct from those in sporadic adult renal neoplasia. Am J Surg Pathol 2006;30:141–53.

20. Taylor KJ, Ramos I, Carter D, et al. Correlation of Doppler US tumor signals with neovascular morphologic features. Radiology 1988;166:57–62.

21. Lee HY, Kim SH, Jung SI, et al. Renal cell carcinoma in an end-stage kidney: evaluation with spectral Doppler ultrasound. J Med Ultrasound 2004;12: 91–4.

22. Silverman SG. What proportion of suspicious-looking renal masses are actually benign? Nat Clin Pract Urol 2007;4:360–1.

23. Frank I, Blute ML, Cheville JC, et al. Solid renal tumors: an analysis of pathological features related to tumor size. J Urol 2003;170:2217–20.

24. Kutikov A, Fossett LK, Ramchandani P, et al. Incidence of benign pathologic findings at partial nephrectomy for solitary renal mass presumed to be renal cell carcinoma on preoperative imaging. Urology 2006;68:737–40.

25. Laguna MP, Kümmerlin I, Rioja J, et al. Biopsy of a renal mass: where are we now? Curr Opin Urol 2009;19:447–53.

Renal Masses as Characterized by Ultrasound Contrast

Michele Bertolotto, MD[a],*, Lorenzo E. Derchi, MD[b],
Calogero Cicero, MD[c], Mariano Iannelli, MD[a]

KEYWORDS

- CEUS • Renal tumors • Renal masses • Characterization • Contrast media • Microbubbles

KEY POINTS

- Contrast-enhanced ultrasound is an emerging technique for the evaluation of renal masses.
- Microbubble contrast agents are safe and not nephrotoxic. Adverse reactions are rare.
- Established applications are differentiation between solid tumors, pseudolesions, and complex cysts; characterization of complex cysts as benign or malignant; and evaluation of tumor ablation.
- Quantitative assessment of lesion perfusion in response to angiosuppressive medications is an emerging application in patients with advanced renal neoplasms.

INTRODUCTION

The widespread use of abdominal imaging for nonurologic complaints has led to a significant increase in the detection of incidental renal masses.[1] Ultrasound is often the first imaging modality. Once identified, lesions are usually categorized and staged on contrast-enhanced computed tomography (CT) or magnetic resonance (MR) imaging.

Contrast-enhanced ultrasound (CEUS) has potential in the categorization of focal renal lesions as well.[2,3] Major advantages of this technique are the possibility of injecting microbubbles without regard for renal function, and the near-total discrimination between contrast and tissue signal enabling clear differentiation between vascularized/vital and nonvascularized/nonviable areas.[4] Adequate evaluation of renal and tumor perfusion is also usually obtained in old, obese, and noncollaborating patients with a spatial resolution approaching that of conventional gray-scale ultrasound imaging. Because microbubble contrast agents are not nephrotoxic, they should be considered in every case if they offer the possibility of achieving enough diagnostic information, particularly in patients with renal impairment, in whom CT or MR imaging should only be used in cases of inconclusive examination and strong clinical need,[5] or for staging after an established diagnosis of neoplasia has been reached.

MICROBUBBLE CONTRAST AGENTS

Ultrasound contrast agents[6] are gas-filled microbubbles with a mean diameter of less than that of a red blood cell (ie, 2–6 μm). They are composed of a shell of biocompatible materials, including proteins, lipids, or biopolymers containing gasses with low solubility and diffusibility such as perfluorocarbon or sulfur hexafluoride. Microbubbles behave as an active source of sound, modifying the characteristic signature of the echo from blood. They are excellent enhancers because acoustic impedance of gas is largely different from that of blood. When properly insonated with a high-power ultrasound beam, microbubbles collapse, producing a high-intensity, broadband transient signal. When the power of the ultrasound beam is lower, microbubbles undergo complex

[a] Department of Radiology, Ospedale di Cattinara, University of Trieste, Strada di Fiume 447, Trieste 34149, Italy; [b] Department of Radiology, University of Genoa, Largo Rosanna Benzi 8, Genova 16132, Italy; [c] Department of Radiology, San Bassiano Hospital, Via Dei Lotti 40, Bassano del Grappa (VI) 36061, Italy
* Corresponding author.
E-mail address: bertolot@units.it

Ultrasound Clin 8 (2013) 581–592
http://dx.doi.org/10.1016/j.cult.2013.07.003
1556-858X/13/$ – see front matter © 2013 Elsevier Inc. All rights reserved.

oscillation and work by resonating, rapidly contracting and expanding in response to the pressure changes of the sound wave. A variety of contrast-specific ultrasound modes has been developed to detect the nonlinear behavior of microbubbles.

Microbubble contrast agents are eliminated through the lungs (ie, breathing) and the liver. They are neither filtered by the kidney nor are able to enter the interstitial spaces. Until metabolized, they act as blood pool agents. The lack of renal excretion explains the absence of kidney toxicity.

STUDY PROCEDURE

CEUS of the kidney is currently performed using low-mechanical-index nondestructive modes in real time.[7] After a preliminary gray-scale and color Doppler evaluation, the ultrasound equipment is set for contrast examination. Nondestructive imaging is typically obtained by setting the mechanical index between 0.2 and 0.06, depending on the equipment used. We use sulfur hexafluoride microbubbles (SonoVue, Bracco Imaging), the only

microbubble contrast agent licensed for general imaging in European countries. Agents licensed in other countries, such as perfluoropropane (Definity, Lantheus Medical Imaging) and perfluorobutane (Sonazoid, Daiichi Sankio), have similar performance in imaging the kidney. In our clinical practice, a microbubble bolus of 1.2 to 2.4 mL is injected to evaluate each kidney using a 20-gauge intravenous cannula, followed by a 10-mL saline flush. According to the guidelines of the European Federation of Societies for Ultrasound in Medicine and Biology (EFSUMB), a real-time video clip should be recorded for review and documentation. The clip should ideally include the whole examination or at least the most relevant parts. If possible, the clip should be stored permanently.[5]

RENAL VASCULAR ANATOMY

Kidney enhances quickly and intensively after microbubble administration (**Fig. 1**). The arterial pedicle and main branches enhance first, followed within few seconds by complete fill-in of the cortex. Unlike Doppler techniques, signal from microbubbles is independent from the angle of

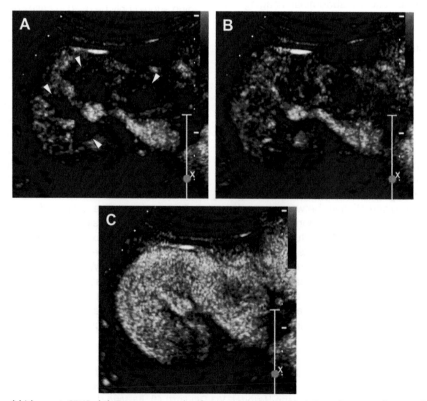

Fig. 1. Normal kidney at CEUS. (*A*) Twenty seconds after microbubble administration, renal parenchyma shows homogeneous enhancement with the exclusion of the medulla (*arrowheads*). (*B*) Thirty seconds after microbubble injection there is filling of the cortex and of the outer portion of the medulla. (*C*) Ninety seconds after the injection there is complete enhancement of the medulla as well.

insonation, and depiction of renal perfusion is also excellent at the renal poles. Medullary vascularization can be evaluated as well. The outer medulla enhances first, followed by gradual fill-in of the pyramids.[7–11] There is no microbubble accumulation in the renal parenchyma. As contrast concentration in the general circulation decreases, enhancement fades.

DIFFERENTIAL DIAGNOSIS BETWEEN CYSTIC AND SOLID LESIONS

Because of its excellent sensitivity, CEUS is highly effective at detecting intralesional flows, and is therefore able to differentiate solid hypovascular tumors from atypical cystic masses (**Fig. 2**).[12,13] Preliminary investigation suggests that CEUS is more sensitive than contrast-enhanced CT in detecting blood flow in hypovascularized lesions.[13,14] CEUS can therefore be used to differentiate hypovascular solid tumors presenting equivocal enhancement on contrast-enhanced CT from avascular renal cysts, which do not display typical ultrasound features (**Fig. 3**).

DIFFERENTIAL DIAGNOSIS BETWEEN SOLID RENAL LESIONS AND PSEUDOTUMORS

Renal pseudotumors, encompassing the column of Bertin and dromedary hump, can often be evaluated with conventional color Doppler ultrasound alone. In some cases, differentiation from tumor is difficult, and recourse to CT and/or MR imaging for confirmation is required. Renal tumors present with different enhancement, compared with healthy parenchyma, in at least one vascular phase. This characteristic allows differential diagnosis between tumors and pseudotumors, the latter presenting with the same enhancing characteristics as the surrounding parenchyma in all vascular phases (**Fig. 4**).[9,10,13,15–17] One potentially helpful application of CEUS is in patients who present with loin pain caused by hemorrhage and in whom there may be a suspicion of an underlying tumor. Often conventional ultrasound shows a large heterogeneous mass. CEUS identifies active bleeding and helps differentiate hematoma from vascularized tumor tissue (**Fig. 5**).

CHARACTERIZATION OF COMPLEX CYSTIC RENAL MASSES

There is increasing clinical evidence that CEUS allows characterization of renal cystic lesions as benign or malignant with at least the same diagnostic accuracy as contrast-enhanced CT (**Fig. 6**). CEUS is more sensitive than CT in detecting enhancement of the cystic wall, septa (**Fig. 7**), and solid components[18]; it depicts more septa than CT, which may appear thicker, resulting in a Bosniak score upgrade.[19] According to Park and colleagues,[20] the diagnostic accuracy in differentiating benign from malignant cystic masses was higher for CEUS compared with CT (90% and 74%, respectively). In 26% of lesions there were differences in the Bosniak score, which was upgraded by CEUS. Moreover, for 6 lesions, solid components were detected by CEUS but not by CT. Ascenti and colleagues[21] prospectively compared 40 consecutive cystic renal masses with CEUS and CT using the Bosniak system. For both CEUS and CT, interobserver agreement was high, and a complete concordance was found between CEUS and CT in the differentiation of surgical and nonsurgical cysts. Presence of wall calcification limits contrast interrogation, resulting in a possible limitation of CEUS for a full evaluation of

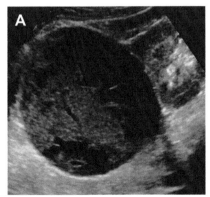 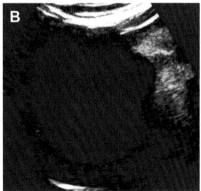

Fig. 2. Complex renal cyst of the right kidney. (*A*) Gray-scale ultrasound shows a renal lesion with inhomogeneous echogenic content that cannot be characterized as solid or cystic. (*B*) CEUS shows lack of enhancement of the lesion, which is characterized by minimal wall enhancement and no irregularities, consistent with a benign, minimally complicated cyst (category II cyst following the Bosniak classification).

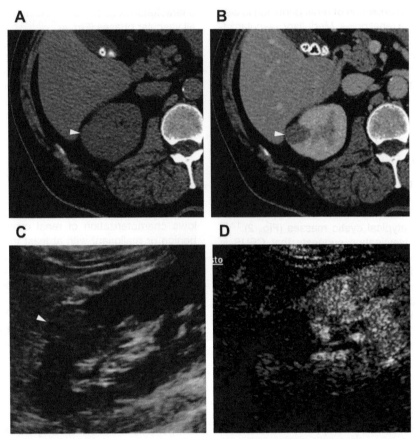

Fig. 3. Equivocal enhancement at CT. Right renal lesion (*arrowhead*) presenting with a density of 30 HU in the unenhanced scan (*A*) and 45 HU on the contrast-enhanced scan (*B*). The lesion (*arrowhead*) is echogenic on gray-scale ultrasound (*C*), and presents with obvious enhancement after microbubble injection (*D*), consistent with solid, hypovascular renal tumor.

the mass only if a significant proportion of the lesion is calcified (**Fig. 8**).

Based on these findings, CEUS should be used to characterize renal masses with a complex cystic appearance, provided that the lesion can be explored adequately. CT may be the standard method still required for staging purpose in patients with malignant cystic lesions. Nevertheless, CEUS is well suited for follow-up of nonsurgical lesions to detect any morphologic changes such as thickening of septa, appearance of a solid nodule, or contrast-enhanced modifications indicating progression of the disease, with the benefits of a reduction of cost and radiation.[22] In the follow-up, the increase of size might not represent a suspicious criterion of progression because benign cysts can also grow.[23]

EVALUATION OF SOLID RENAL LESIONS

Early investigations dealt with differentiation of renal tumors, particularly angiomyolipoma and

renal cell carcinomas, by means of different features of time-intensity curves after microbubble bolus injection, with early washout, heterogeneous enhancement, and enhanced peritumoural rim all features on CEUS that were strongly associated with carcinoma. However, renal cancer does not show a typical perfusion pattern at CEUS.[24] It usually shows diffuse homogeneous or heterogeneous enhancement during the early corticomedullary phase, often with a hypervascular appearance, and has variable enhancement in the remaining phases. Enhancement is limited to the solid viable regions, sparing intratumoral avascular necrotic, hemorrhagic, or cystic components (**Fig. 9**).[9,25] Some lesions, usually papillary or chromophobe tumors but also metastases and approximately 13% to 15% of clear cell carcinomas, enhance less than the surrounding parenchyma in all vascular phases.[26] Compared with large lesions, small tumors more often present with homogeneous contrast enhancement.[27] According to the EFSUMB guidelines, CEUS is not

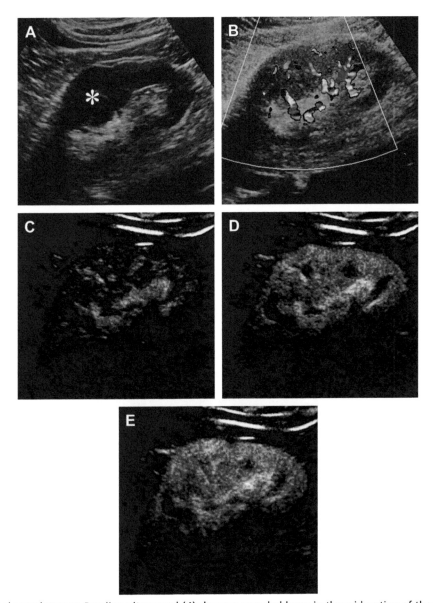

Fig. 4. Renal pseudotumor. Baseline ultrasound (*A*) shows a rounded lump in the midportion of the left kidney (*asterisk*) suggesting a renal tumor. Color Doppler interrogation (*B*) does not allow further characterization of the lump. CEUS scans obtained 20 seconds (*C*), 35 seconds (*D*), and 90 seconds (*E*) after microbubble injection reveal identical enhancement of the lump and of the renal parenchyma in all the vascular phases.

able to differentiate between malignant and benign solid masses.[5] A confident diagnosis of angiomyolipoma, in particular, is only reached by documenting the presence of fat within the lesion with CT or MR imaging.

Renal cell carcinomas generally do not have a histologic capsule. A pseudocapsule may be identified resulting from tumor growth producing ischemia and necrosis of adjacent normal parenchyma. This feature is not described in the tumor-node-metastasis classification but is a pathologic feature frequently seen in early-stage,

low-grade carcinomas. Ascenti and colleagues[28] investigated the ability of CEUS to detect a pseudocapsule in 32 patients with 40 renal masses, which were identified in 12 of 14 pathologically proven cases. Jiang and colleagues[27] correlated CEUS features of 92 pathologically confirmed clear cell renal cell carcinomas in relation to tumor size. In patients with tumors less than or equal to 2 cm, a pseudocapsule appeared in 3 of 13 cases (23%); in tumors from 2 to 5 cm, in 38 of 58 cases (66%); and in tumors larger than 5 cm, in 5 of 21 cases (24%).

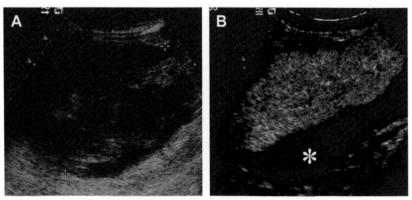

Fig. 5. Patient presenting with palpable right renal lump following a minor abdominal trauma. (A) Gray-scale ultrasound showing an inhomogeneous lump suggesting an underlying tumor. (B) CEUS shows normal kidney and large subcapsular hematoma (*asterisk*).

According to Ignee and colleagues,[29] CEUS is able to identify renal vein invasion in patients with solid renal lesions with an accuracy that is at least comparable with contrast-enhanced CT, and to differentiate appositional thrombus from tumor tissue thrombosis (**Fig. 10**).

PERCUTANEOUS ABLATION THERAPIES

Even though nephron-sparing surgery is the standard of care for small, localized renal tumors, alternative minimally invasive options, such as radiofrequency ablation and cryoablation, are indicated in selected patients with comorbidities or

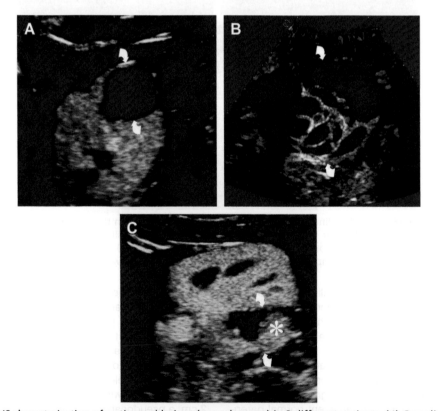

Fig. 6. CEUS characterization of cystic renal lesions (*curved arrows*) in 3 different patients. (A) Complicated, presumably benign, cyst requiring follow-up because of slightly thickened enhancing wall with no irregularities. (B) Indeterminate renal lesion that requires surgical removal because of multiple thick irregular septa, and thick enhancing wall. (C) Overtly malignant cystic tumor with enhancing tumor vegetation (*asterisk*).

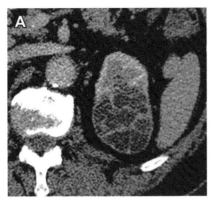
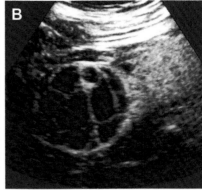

Fig. 7. Complex cyst in the left kidney. (A) Contrast-enhanced CT shows a left renal cyst presenting with barely enhancing thin septa and slightly enhancing wall. The lesion is characterized as a category IIF cyst according to the Bosniak criteria. (B) CEUS showing obvious enhancement of the wall and septa.

reduced life expectancy. There is increasing evidence that CEUS is a reproducible technique with high predictive values and specificity for early detection of residual tumor after ablation.[30–34] However, sensitivity is lower than with CT/MR imaging.[31] There is an excellent correlation between the ablation volume measured with CEUS and pathologically.[35] Successful ablation is depicted as an area lacking contrast enhancement (Fig. 11). Early after the ablation, peripheral reactive hyperemia may be misinterpreted as residual tumor. Meticulous comparison with preprocedural examinations and evaluation of lesion morphology are of paramount importance to avoid misdiagnosis, because residual tumor presents as a nodular or crescentlike area with kinetics and morphologic characteristics of enhancement reflecting those observed in the tumor before the treatment (Fig. 12).[31]

Most investigations deal with the use of CEUS to monitor the results of radiofrequency ablation

of renal tumors.[30–32] A recent pilot study investigated the use of CEUS compared with CT/MR before (n = 26), 3 months (n = 32), and 12 months (n = 21) after laparoscopic renal cryoablation. Results showed high concordance between CT/MR and CEUS.[34] Likewise, in another series of 42 patients, high concordance was found between CEUS and CT/MR before and after tumor cryoablation.[36] In our series of 29 patients with 30 lesions, CEUS performed less than 48 hours after percutaneous renal tumor cryoablation was able to identify residual disease in 1 case, and to address the issue of another ablation treatment.

MONITORING ANGIOSUPPRESSIVE THERAPIES IN ADVANCED DISEASE

The treatment of metastatic renal cell carcinoma remains problematic. Chemotherapy and radiation do not improve prognosis substantially. Cytokine immunotherapies such as high-dose interleukin 2

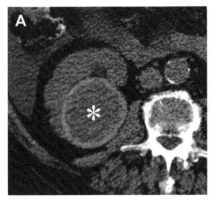
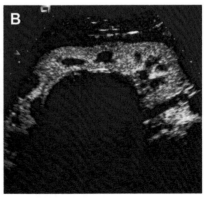

Fig. 8. Limitations of CEUS in characterization of cystic renal lesions. (A) Unenhanced CT showing a cyst in the right kidney (asterisk) with hyperdense wall by presence of thin wall calcifications. (B) Acoustic shadow produced by the wall hampers evaluation of the lesion content at CEUS.

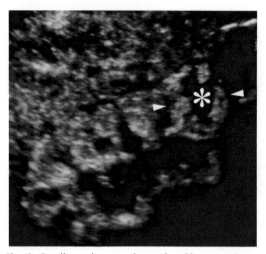

Fig. 9. Small renal tumor (*arrowheads*) presenting a viable peripheral portion and a central avascular necrotic region (*asterisk*).

or interferon alfa work effectively only in a minority of patients. As many as 90% of clear cell renal cell carcinomas contain mutations located in the von Hippel-Lindau tumor suppressor gene, which eventually result in increased expression of hypoxia-inducible genes, including vascular endothelial growth factor (VEGF). VEGF activates tumor angiogenesis and promotes metastatic tumor spread. Histopathologic evaluations reveal that clear cell renal cell carcinoma is a highly vascularized neoplasm with evidence of abundant angiogenesis and abnormal blood vessel development, which are the grounds for use of VEGF-targeted angiosuppressive therapies, such as VEGF neutralizing antibody and VEGF receptor tyrosine kinase inhibitors, in metastatic clear cell renal carcinoma. The introduction into clinical practice of these therapeutic strategies raises concern for identification of adequate imaging procedures. The Response Evaluation Criteria in Solid Tumors (RECIST), used to assess conventional cytotoxic chemotherapy, do not effectively evaluate angiosuppressive therapies, because lesions

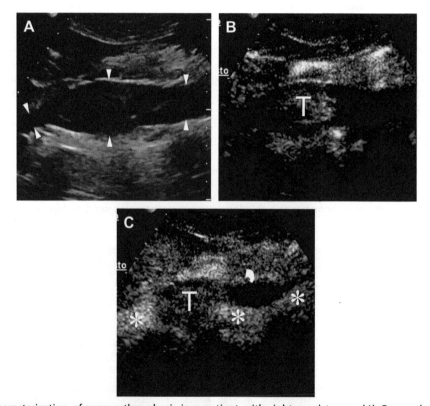

Fig. 10. Characterization of venous thrombosis in a patient with right renal tumor. (*A*) Gray-scale ultrasound showing extensive thrombosis within the inferior vena cava (*arrowheads*). (*B*) CEUS image obtained 12 seconds after microbubble injection showing neoplastic thrombosis, presenting with enhancement of the tumor thrombus (T). (*C*) CEUS obtained 49 seconds after microbubble injection shows washout in the tumor thrombus (T), microbubbles in the patent portions of the inferior vena cava (*asterisk*), and lack of enhancement in the thrombotic appositional thrombus (*curved arrow*).

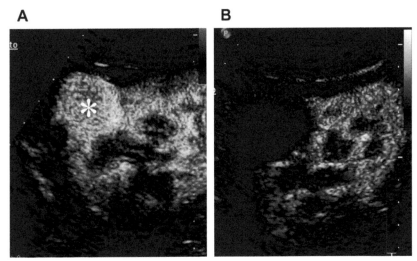

Fig. 11. Successful cryoablation of renal tumor. (A) CEUS of the right kidney shows a homogeneous enhancing renal tumor (*asterisk*). The lesion is completely avascular 24 hours following cryoablation (B), indicating complete ablation of the tumor tissue.

often show little change in size despite substantial clinical benefit. Criteria that additionally take into account lesion vascular changes help to identify patients who show clinical benefit earlier than with using RECIST criteria.[37] CEUS can be used to quantify lesion enhancement changes in response to antiangiogenic treatment. In a preliminary study on patients with metastatic renal cell carcinoma evaluated with CEUS before and after 2 weeks of treatment with sunitinib, a multitargeted receptor tyrosine kinase inhibitor, median tumor fractional blood volume decreased markedly in response to treatment. The investigators concluded that CEUS provides reproducible and sensitive assessment of vascular changes in response to antiangiogenic therapy.[38]

FUSION IMAGING

As mentioned earlier, CEUS can be used as a problem-solving method in characterization of lesions presenting with equivocal appearance on CT or MR imaging. However, especially in cases of small or multifocal lesions, ultrasound lesion identification for target contrast investigation can be difficult and time consuming. A recent pilot

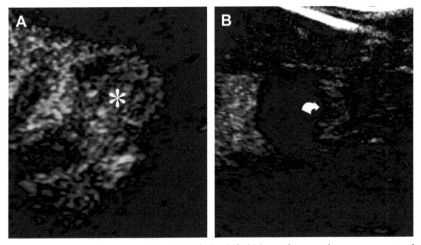

Fig. 12. Incomplete tumor cryoablation. (A) CEUS of the left kidney shows a homogeneous enhancing renal tumor (*asterisk*). (B) A crescentlike enhancing tumor region (*curved arrow*) is recognized 24 hours following cryoablation, consistent with residual viable tumor. After additional cryoablation, CEUS and contrast CT showed an absence of residual tumor tissue (not shown).

study suggested that better results may be obtained with regard to identifying lesions by using CEUS with the image fusion mode, and that operator dependence may be reduced.[39] Limitations include larger expenditure of time, and the need to perform CEUS with the patient in a supine position, to mimic the CT or MR imaging setting and obtain a good registration of the data sets.

INTRAOPERATIVE APPLICATIONS

Partial nephrectomy is traditionally performed with clamping of the hilar vessels to enable an adequate resection margin and lessen blood loss during surgery. Avoiding global ischemia is an emerging concept during the intervention because ischemia time, if prolonged, can be detrimental to the functional recovery of the kidney. Several techniques have been described to assist in zero-ischemia partial nephrectomy wherein selective arterial clamping or ligation is performed of the vessels feeding the tumor. A preliminary investigation on 5 patients showed that CEUS has the potential to intraoperatively monitor in real time the effectiveness of selective devascularization during robot-assisted partial nephrectomy.[40]

SAFETY ISSUES

In theory, interaction of diagnostic ultrasound and contrast agents can produce in vitro bioeffects: cell sonoporation, hemolysis, and cell death. Despite extensive investigations,[41–44] these effects have not been observed in clinical practice. The most common general adverse events reported, occurring in approximately 2% of patients, are the same as those seen with other types of contrast media: headache, warm sensation, and flushing. More unusual events, occurring in less than 1% of patients, are nausea and vomiting, dizziness, chills and fever, altered taste, abdominal pain, respiratory disorders, pharyngitis, pruritus, rash, abnormal vision, dry mouth, personality disorder, insomnia, nervousness, hyperglycemia, peripheral edema, ecchymosis, and sensory-motor paresis. Such effects are usually transient and mild, were also observed in placebo groups, and are similar for many agents. Rare cases suggesting hypersensitivity, which could include skin erythema, bradycardia, hypotension, or anaphylactic shock, have been reported in temporal association with the use of microbubble contrast agents. In a large retrospective analysis of the safety of SonoVue, in more than 23,000 patients the overall reporting rate of serious adverse events was 0.0086% (2 serious adverse events and no deaths).[45] Several other investigations confirm these data.[46–49]

SUMMARY

CEUS is extensively used for nonhepatic applications in many European countries. Several indications for the use of microbubble contrast agents in imaging the kidney are well delineated in the EF-SUMB guidelines,[5] regarding evaluation of focal renal abnormalities, and postprocedural monitoring of ablative procedures. Many of them are discussed in this article. Other potential applications include renal time-intensity curves for objective evaluation of renal and lesion perfusion.

REFERENCES

1. Kane CJ, Mallin K, Ritchey J, et al. Renal cell cancer stage migration: analysis of the National Cancer Data Base. Cancer 2008;113(1):78–83.
2. Bertolotto M, Catalano O. Contrast-enhanced ultrasound: past, present, and future. Ultrasound Clin 2009;4(3):339–67.
3. Barozzi L, Valentino M, Bertolotto M, et al. Contrast enhanced ultrasound of renal diseases. Arch Ital Urol Androl 2010;82(4):232–7.
4. Bertolotto M, Martegani A, Aiani L, et al. Value of contrast-enhanced ultrasonography for detecting renal infarcts proven by contrast enhanced CT. A feasibility study. Eur Radiol 2008;18(2):376–83.
5. Piscaglia F, Nolsoe C, Dietrich CF, et al. The EF-SUMB Guidelines and Recommendations on the Clinical Practice of Contrast Enhanced Ultrasound (CEUS): update 2011 on non-hepatic applications. Ultraschall Med 2012;33(1):33–59.
6. Dalla Palma L, Bertolotto M. Introduction to ultrasound contrast agents: physics overview. Eur Radiol 1999;9(Suppl 3):S338–42.
7. Siracusano S, Bertolotto M, Ciciliato S, et al. The current role of contrast-enhanced ultrasound (CEUS) imaging in the evaluation of renal pathology. World J Urol 2011;29(5):633–8.
8. Tsuruoka K, Yasuda T, Koitabashi K, et al. Evaluation of renal microcirculation by contrast-enhanced ultrasound with sonazoid™ as a contrast agent. Comparison between normal subjects and patients with chronic kidney disease. Int Heart J 2010;51(3):176–82.
9. Correas JM, Claudon M, Tranquart F, et al. The kidney: imaging with microbubble contrast agents. Ultrasound Q 2006;22(1):53–66.
10. Setola SV, Catalano O, Sandomenico F, et al. Contrast-enhanced sonography of the kidney. Abdom Imaging 2007;32(1):21–8.
11. McArthur C, Baxter GM. Current and potential renal applications of contrast-enhanced ultrasound. Clin Radiol 2012;67(9):909–22.

12. Weskott HP. Emerging roles for contrast-enhanced ultrasound. Clin Hemorheol Microcirc 2008;40(1): 51–71.

13. Robbin ML, Lockhart ME, Barr RG. Renal imaging with ultrasound contrast: current status. Radiol Clin North Am 2003;41(5):963–78.

14. Tamai H, Takiguchi Y, Oka M, et al. Contrast-enhanced ultrasonography in the diagnosis of solid renal tumors. J Ultrasound Med 2005;24(12):1635–40.

15. Nilsson A. Contrast-enhanced ultrasound of the kidneys. Eur Radiol 2004;14(Suppl 8):P104–9.

16. Mazziotti S, Zimbaro F, Pandolfo A, et al. Usefulness of contrast-enhanced ultrasonography in the diagnosis of renal pseudotumors. Abdom Imaging 2010;35(2):241–5.

17. Ignee A, Straub B, Schuessler G, et al. Contrast enhanced ultrasound of renal masses. World J Radiol 2010;2(1):15–31.

18. Quaia E, Bertolotto M, Cioffi V, et al. Comparison of contrast-enhanced sonography with unenhanced sonography and contrast-enhanced CT in the diagnosis of malignancy in complex cystic renal masses. AJR Am J Roentgenol 2008;191(4):1239–49.

19. Clevert DA, Minaifar N, Weckbach S, et al. Multislice computed tomography versus contrast-enhanced ultrasound in evaluation of complex cystic renal masses using the Bosniak classification system. Clin Hemorheol Microcirc 2008;39(1–4):171–8.

20. Park BK, Kim B, Kim SH, et al. Assessment of cystic renal masses based on Bosniak classification: comparison of CT and contrast-enhanced US. Eur J Radiol 2007;61(2):310–4.

21. Ascenti G, Mazziotti S, Zimbaro G, et al. Complex cystic renal masses: characterization with contrast-enhanced US. Radiology 2007;243(1):158–65.

22. Nicolau C, Bunesch L, Sebastia C. Renal complex cysts in adults: contrast-enhanced ultrasound. Abdom Imaging 2011;36(6):742–52.

23. Silverman SG, Israel GM, Herts BR, et al. Management of the incidental renal mass. Radiology 2008; 249(1):16–31.

24. Haendl T, Strobel D, Legal W, et al. Renal cell cancer does not show a typical perfusion pattern in contrast-enhanced ultrasound. Ultraschall Med 2009;30(1):58–63 [in German].

25. Siracusano S, Quaia E, Bertolotto M, et al. The application of ultrasound contrast agents in the characterization of renal tumors. World J Urol 2004;22(5): 316–22.

26. Xu ZF, Xu HX, Xie XY, et al. Renal cell carcinoma: real-time contrast-enhanced ultrasound findings. Abdom Imaging 2010;35(6):750–6.

27. Jiang J, Chen Y, Zhou Y, et al. Clear cell renal cell carcinoma: contrast-enhanced ultrasound features relation to tumor size. Eur J Radiol 2010;73(1):162–7.

28. Ascenti G, Gaeta M, Magno C, et al. Contrast-enhanced second-harmonic sonography in the detection of pseudocapsule in renal cell carcinoma. AJR Am J Roentgenol 2004;182(6):1525–30.

29. Ignee A, Straub B, Brix D, et al. The value of contrast enhanced ultrasound (CEUS) in the characterisation of patients with renal masses. Clin Hemorheol Microcirc 2010;46(4):275–90.

30. Meloni MF, Bertolotto M, Alberzoni C, et al. Follow-up after percutaneous radiofrequency ablation of renal cell carcinoma: contrast-enhanced sonography versus contrast-enhanced CT or MRI. AJR Am J Roentgenol 2008;191(4):1233–8.

31. Hoeffel C, Pousset M, Timsit MO, et al. Radiofrequency ablation of renal tumours: diagnostic accuracy of contrast-enhanced ultrasound for early detection of residual tumour. Eur Radiol 2010; 20(8):1812–21.

32. Kong WT, Zhang WW, Guo HQ, et al. Application of contrast-enhanced ultrasonography after radiofrequency ablation for renal cell carcinoma: is it sufficient for assessment of therapeutic response? Abdom Imaging 2011;36(3):342–7.

33. Wink MH, Lagerveld BW, Laguna MP, et al. Cryotherapy for renal-cell cancer: diagnosis, treatment, and contrast-enhanced ultrasonography for follow-up. J Endourol 2006;20(7):456–8 [discussion: 458–9].

34. Barwari K, Wijkstra H, van Delden OM, et al. Contrast-enhanced ultrasound for the evaluation of the cryolesion after laparoscopic renal cryoablation: an initial report. J Endourol 2013;27(4):402–7.

35. Slabaugh TK, Machaidze Z, Hennigar R, et al. Monitoring radiofrequency renal lesions in real time using contrast-enhanced ultrasonography: a porcine model. J Endourol 2005;19(5):579–83.

36. Liu HM, Zhao SL, Qu LX, et al. Value of contrast-enhanced ultrasound imaging in monitoring malignant tumor during argon-helium cryosurgery. Nan fang yi ke da xue xue bao 2011;31(9):1622–5 [in Chinese].

37. Bertolotto M, Pozzato G, Croce LS, et al. Blood flow changes in hepatocellular carcinoma after the administration of thalidomide assessed by reperfusion kinetics during microbubble infusion: preliminary results. Invest Radiol 2006;41(1):15–21.

38. Williams R, Hudson JM, Lloyd BA, et al. Dynamic microbubble contrast-enhanced US to measure tumor response to targeted therapy: a proposed clinical protocol with results from renal cell carcinoma patients receiving antiangiogenic therapy. Radiology 2011;260(2):581–90.

39. Helck A, D'Anastasi M, Notohamiprodjo M, et al. Multimodality imaging using ultrasound image fusion in renal lesions. Clin Hemorheol Microcirc 2012;50(1–2):79–89.

40. Rao AR, Gray R, Mayer E, et al. Occlusion angiography using intraoperative contrast-enhanced ultrasound scan (CEUS): a novel technique

demonstrating segmental renal blood supply to assist zero-ischaemia robot-assisted partial nephrectomy. Eur Urol 2013;63(5):913–9.

41. Morel DR, Schwieger I, Hohn L, et al. Human pharmacokinetics and safety evaluation of SonoVue, a new contrast agent for ultrasound imaging. Invest Radiol 2000;35(1):80–5.

42. Myreng Y, Molstad P, Ytre-Arne K, et al. Safety of the transpulmonary ultrasound contrast agent NC100100: a clinical and haemodynamic evaluation in patients with suspected or proved coronary artery disease. Heart 1999;82(3):333–5.

43. Robbin ML, Eisenfeld AJ. Perflenapent emulsion: a US contrast agent for diagnostic radiology– multicenter, double-blind comparison with a placebo. EchoGen Contrast Ultrasound Study Group. Radiology 1998;207(3):717–22.

44. Borges AC, Walde T, Reibis RK, et al. Does contrast echocardiography with Optison induce myocardial necrosis in humans? J Am Soc Echocardiogr 2002; 15(10 Pt 1):1080–6.

45. Piscaglia F, Bolondi L. The safety of Sonovue in abdominal applications: retrospective analysis of 23188 investigations. Ultrasound Med Biol 2006; 32(9):1369–75.

46. Aggeli C, Felekos I, Siasos G, et al. Ultrasound contrast agents: updated data on safety profile. Curr Pharm Des 2012;18(15):2253–8.

47. Gabriel RS, Smyth YM, Menon V, et al. Safety of ultrasound contrast agents in stress echocardiography. Am J Cardiol 2008;102(9):1269–72.

48. Dijkmans PA, Juffermans LJ, van Dijk J, et al. Safety and feasibility of real time adenosine myocardial contrast echocardiography with emphasis on induction of arrhythmias: a study in healthy volunteers and patients with stable coronary artery disease. Echocardiography 2009;26(7):807–14.

49. Aggeli C, Giannopoulos G, Roussakis G, et al. Safety of myocardial flash-contrast echocardiography in combination with dobutamine stress testing for the detection of ischaemia in 5250 studies. Heart 2008;94(12):1571–7.

Vascular Complications of Renal Transplant

Mehmet Ruhi Onur, MD[a],*, Vikram Dogra, MD[b]

KEYWORDS

- Renal transplantation • Vascular complications • Ultrasound • Doppler

KEY POINTS

- Renal transplant provides much longer survival than hemodialysis and peritoneal dialysis for patients with end-stage kidney disease.
- Prevention of complications in recipients improves survival rates.
- Imaging studies are crucial for early recognition of vascular complications of renal transplant.
- Ultrasound is the key imaging method in the evaluation of renal transplants in the immediate postoperative period and the long-term follow-up.
- Color flow Doppler ultrasound depicts most vascular complications.

INTRODUCTION

Renal transplantation is the choice of treatment in patients with end-stage renal disease. It is a cost-effective treatment method compared with hemodialysis or peritoneal dialysis with the advantages of better long-term survival and a better quality of life for patients.[1] Continued improvements in renal graft survival is based on refined surgical techniques, continuous progress in immunosuppressive therapy as well as early detection of complications. Despite the improvements in surgical techniques, vascular complications occur in 1% to 2% of renal transplants.[2] Vascular complications can be classified as graft renal artery stenosis or thrombosis, graft renal vein stenosis (RVS) or thrombosis, arteriovenous fistula, intrarenal and extrarenal pseudoaneurysm, arterial kinking, allograft torsion, and infarction. Ultrasound is the mainstay imaging technique in the evaluation of renal transplant. Gray-scale, color flow, and spectral Doppler ultrasound are routinely used in the detection of the complications to prevent irreversible changes and graft dysfunction. This article aims to illustrate the imaging findings of vascular complications of the renal transplant and highlight the role of ultrasound in early detection and management of these complications.

VASCULAR ANATOMY OF RENAL TRANSPLANT

Accurate sonographic evaluation of renal transplant depends on awareness of surgical anatomy of the transplant. The transplant kidney can be implanted either extraperitoneally or intraperitoneally in the right or left iliac fossa. Right iliac fossa extraperitoneal placement is preferred.

In cadaveric kidney transplantation, end-to-side anastomosis to the external iliac vasculature is the most frequently preferred arterial anastomosis technique.[3] Cadaveric kidneys usually have intact main renal artery with an attached portion of the aorta. The aorta portion can be trimmed to an oval configuration (Carrel patch) and anastomosed to the external iliac artery in an end-to-side fashion.[4] In living donor transplantation, end-to-side anastomosis of the donor renal artery to the

Financial Disclosure and/or Conflicts of Interest: The authors have nothing to disclose.
[a] Department of Radiology, Faculty of Medicine, University of Firat, Firat Universitesi Hastanesi, Rektorluk Kampusu, Elazig 23119, Turkey; [b] Department of Imaging Sciences, Faculty of Medicine, University of Rochester, 601 Elmwood Avenue, Rochester, NY 1462, USA
* Corresponding author.
E-mail address: ruhionur@yahoo.com

recipient external iliac artery or end-to-end anastomosis to the recipient internal iliac artery may be performed.[3] Anastomosis of the venous vasculature is always performed as end-to-side anastomosis to the recipient external iliac vein at either cadaveric or living donor transplantation. Approximately 20% of renal transplants require multiple arterial or venous anastomoses.[5]

IMAGING TECHNIQUES IN VASCULAR COMPLICATIONS OF RENAL TRANSPLANT
Ultrasonography

Gray-scale ultrasound
Ultrasound is the first imaging technique in the postoperative evaluation and long-term follow-up of the renal transplant. Relatively low cost, lack of ionizing radiation, portability, and ease of use are the main advantages of ultrasound in the evaluation of the renal transplant. A baseline ultrasound with color flow and spectral Doppler ultrasound within the first 24 to 48 hours is recommended to detect early complications of the renal transplant. The transplant kidney has a similar appearance to native kidney on gray-scale ultrasound. Renal pyramids appear more hypoechoic relative to renal parenchyma in the transplant kidney. The superficial localization of transplant kidney makes interpretation of transplant kidney easier than native kidney. High-frequency transducers used in the sonographic examination of transplant kidney provide high-resolution scanning.

Color flow and power Doppler ultrasound
Color flow Doppler ultrasound is a reliable, noninvasive, and easily available imaging technique that demonstrates the vasculature of the graft, transplant perfusion, and recipient's iliac vessels. Color flow Doppler evaluation steps of renal transplant vasculature include assessment of the recipient's iliac artery and vein, arterial and venous anastomosis, main transplant artery and vein, and intrarenal vessels. In a well-perfused kidney arcuate arteries and sometimes the interlobular arteries should be filled with color on color flow Doppler ultrasound. However visualization of the flow in the vessels on color flow Doppler ultrasound is not sufficient to make a decision about the outcome of the transplant. Spectral Doppler ultrasound of segmental and interlobar vessels reveals fast systolic upstroke with a subsequent slow decay in diastole similar to native kidney.[6] Transplant renal arteries may manifest with marked tortuosity, which necessitates accurate Doppler angle correction during velocity measurement.

Assessment of intrarenal vasculature with color flow Doppler ultrasound can be performed with low wall filter to visualize slow flow in the intrarenal vessels.[7] Abnormal findings in intrarenal color flow Doppler ultrasound examination may represent complications of main or intrarenal arteries. Spectral Doppler ultrasound including quantitative indices such as peak systolic velocity (PSV) of the transplant renal artery, PSV ratio of the transplant renal artery to the iliac artery, resistive index (RI), pulsatility index, acceleration time, and acceleration index of the intrarenal arteries are necessary to determine the possible vascular abnormalities of the renal transplant (**Fig. 1**). In healthy renal transplants, intrarenal arteries exhibit low resistance and fast acceleration with early systolic peak on spectral Doppler ultrasound.[8] The intrarenal veins manifest monophasic waveform with low velocity.[7] An elevated RI (>0.8) on spectral Doppler ultrasound suggests renal transplant dysfunction.[3] However the specificity of RI in renal transplant dysfunction is low. A threshold level of 0.9 was reported to have 43% sensitivity and 67% specificity.[9] Power Doppler ultrasound demonstrates perfusion of the transplant kidney. The sensitivity of power Doppler in the detection of the vascular changes of graft dysfunction is higher than RI evaluation.[10] Alterations in the small vessels of the renal transplant can be accurately evaluated with power Doppler ultrasound.

B-Flow ultrasound
B-flow ultrasound has greater spatial and temporal resolution than color Doppler imaging. Clearer definition of the transplant vessels can be achieved by B-flow ultrasound. B-flow ultrasound was found to be useful in the evaluation of renal vascular anastomotic stenoses.[11]

Contrast-enhanced ultrasound
Contrast-enhanced ultrasound can assess the renal allograft perfusion both qualitatively and quantitatively. Microbubbles used in ultrasound contrast materials improve the detection and characterization of renal perfusion abnormalities. Transplant kidneys manifest with complete enhancement 10 to 20 seconds after microbubble injection.[12] New ultrasound technologies such as pulse inversion harmonic and coded harmonic imaging techniques using ultrasound contrast agents demonstrate very slow flow without Doppler artifacts.[3] Global perfusion status and focal perfusion defects in transplant kidneys can be depicted more accurately by these techniques.[13] Harmonic sonography with a microbubble contrast agent was found to have good correlation with technetium-99 diethylene triamine penta acetic acid renal perfusion images in terms of detecting renal perfusion abnormalities.[13]

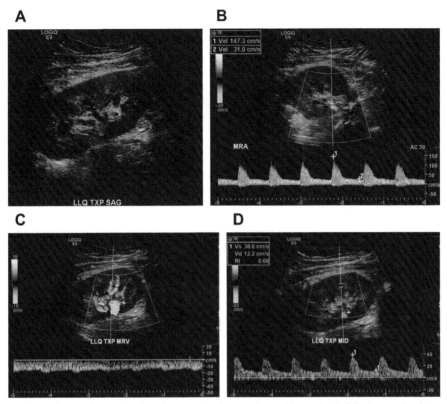

Fig. 1. Gray-scale and color flow Doppler ultrasound of normal renal transplant. (*A*) Gray-scale ultrasound demonstrates a transplant kidney with normal appearance. (*B*) Color flow Doppler ultrasound reveals low resistance flow within the transplant renal artery. (*C*) Color flow Doppler ultrasound demonstrates venous flow in the transplant renal vein. (*D*) Spectral Doppler ultrasound reveals vascular flow with low resistance (RI: 0.68) in the interlobar artery.

Computed Tomography

Multidetector computed tomography (MDCT) is a way of noninvasive imaging to demonstrate vascular complications of transplant kidney. Multiplanar imaging capability of MDCT may reveal the site and degree of abnormality of the transplant vasculature. Less volume of iodinized contrast media is required in MDCT angiography than digital subtraction angiography (DSA).[14] MDCT angiography may demonstrate the stenosis in the recipient's iliac vessels, which can mimic transplant renal artery stenosis (TRAS).

Magnetic Resonance Imaging

Magnetic resonance (MR) angiography may be used to recognize vascular complications of renal transplant. The absence of ionizing radiation, iodinated contrast, or arterial catheterization is a major advantage of MR imaging in the evaluation of renal transplant. MR angiography has evolved as a useful imaging technique especially in the evaluation of vascular stenosis.[15]

Nuclear Imaging

Radionuclide images provide morphologic and functional assessment in the evaluation of renal transplants. Perfusion of renal transplant can be qualitatively interpreted by radionuclide imaging. Administration of angiotensin-converting enzyme inhibitors is helpful to evaluate TRAS. Technetium-99 diethylene triamine penta acetic acid is used to evaluate renal perfusion and perfusion defects.[1]

DSA

DSA is the gold standard technique in the diagnosis of vascular complications of renal transplant. However DSA is rarely preferred due to the possible harmful effects of iodinized contrast media. DSA may be helpful in the localization of the vascular complication. MR angiography and MDCT angiography has replaced DSA in clinical situations when color flow Doppler ultrasound demonstrates positive findings. Groin hematoma, renal artery dissection, thrombosis, perforation, and acute kidney injury secondary to contrast-induced nephropathy can occur after DSA in renal transplant patients.[4]

VASCULAR COMPLICATIONS
Renal Artery Stenosis

TRAS constitutes 75% of vascular complications of renal transplant with an occurrence rate of 3% to 12% in patients following renal transplantation.[4,14,16–18] Predisposing factors for TRAS are cadaveric transplant, end-to-end anastomosis, surgical clamp injury, intimal dissection, inadequate suturing technique, long or kinking artery, prolonged cold ischemia time, acute cellular rejection, and cytomegalovirus infection.[19] The risk of TRAS is 3-fold in patients with end-to-end anastomoses than end-to-side anastomoses.[20]

TRAS may present as early TRAS or late TRAS in the period between 3 months and 2 years after transplantation, respectively.[21] Early TRAS may occur within a week after renal transplantation secondary to intimal dissection, imperfect suturing technique of the anastomosis, and kinking of the graft artery.[22] TRAS usually occurs in the anastomosis site.[23] Other localizations of stenosis include artery segments proximal to the anastomosis and distal to the anastomosis. Anastomotic stenosis usually results from vessel perfusion injury, faulty surgical technique, or reaction to suture material. The stenosis on the proximal donor artery arises from the intimal injury caused during organ retrieval. Proximal TRAS occurs in up to 2.4% of patients mostly 1 year after transplantation.[4] Pseudo TRAS is described by stenosis in the native iliac arteries of the transplant secondary to preexisting or developing atherosclerotic changes or intimal injury resulting from organ retrieval or diminished perfusion.[23] Diffuse stenosis of the artery was reported to be related to immunologic disorders of the vascular endothelium or cytomegalovirus infection. Stenosis of more than 50% of renal artery results in significant hemodynamic changes.[23] Presenting symptoms of TRAS in the immediate period are oliguria or anuria. After the first week, refractory hypertension may occur. The presence of only moderate hypertension in the transplant recipients is not a reliable indicator of TRAS because it may be observed in 65% of transplant recipients.[3] Rarely, TRAS is asymptomatic. Graft dysfunction may also result from TRAS. Iliac artery stenosis may mimic TRAS but patients with iliac artery stenosis have a weak femoral pulse.[23]

Gray-scale ultrasound reveals focal luminal narrowing, mural thickening, and mural calcification in the renal artery.[10] Color flow Doppler ultrasound should be the initial imaging technique in the evaluation of TRAS. The sensitivity and specificity of Doppler ultrasound in the detection of TRAS range between 87%–94% and 86%–100%, respectively.[24] MR angiography, computed tomography angiography, and radionuclide imaging (captopril scan) can also be used in the diagnosis of TRAS.

Extrarenal and intrarenal color flow and spectral Doppler ultrasound findings in TRAS are summarized in **Tables 1** and **2**, respectively.[1] Color flow Doppler ultrasound demonstrates color aliasing at the stenotic site secondary to increased flow velocity. Suggestive findings of hemodynamically significant stenosis are a PSV of more than 200 to 250 cm/s and the ratio of PSV in the transplant main renal artery and external iliac artery of more than 1.8.[23] Peak systolic velocity greater than 200 cm/s depicts TRAS with 90% sensitivity and 87.5% specificity.[25] Baxter and colleagues[26] reported 100% sensitivity and 95% specificity in the detection of TRAS by using 250 cm/s as a threshold PSV. In asymptomatic transplant patients, 300 cm/s was suggested as the threshold value in the depiction of TRAS (**Fig. 2**).[27] Elevated PSV with normal and stable RI suggests postoperative physiologic adaptation, which can be encountered between the posttransplant immediate period to 1 to 3 months after transplantation (**Fig. 3**).[28] In addition to velocity changes, marked distal turbulence resulting in spectral broadening can be observed in spectral Doppler ultrasound. Observation of aliasing indicates severe stenosis of more than 80%.[8]

Assessment of intrarenal waveforms provides indirect evidence suggesting TRAS. Evaluation of intrarenal arteries should include at least one interlobar artery from the upper and lower poles and interpolar segments of the transplant kidney. In TRAS, color flow Doppler ultrasound demonstrates flattening of the systolic peak and tardus-parvus waveform in intrarenal interlobar and arcuate arteries. Prolonged acceleration time (time from the start of the systole to systolic peak), diminished acceleration index (slope of

Table 1		
Extrarenal spectral Doppler ultrasound findings in TRAS		
Extrarenal Parameters		**Values**
Peak systolic velocity		>250 cm/s
PSV RA at stenosis/PSV external iliac artery		>1.8
Velocity gradient between stenotic and prestenotic segments		>2

Table 2
Intrarenal spectral Doppler ultrasound findings in TRAS

Intrarenal Parameter	Value
Resistive index	<0.6
Pulsatility index	<1.2
Acceleration time	$\geq$100 ms
Acceleration index	<300 cm/s^2

the systolic uptake), and loss of a normal early systolic compliance peak constitute intrarenal vasculature findings of TRAS.[29] When the extrarenal and intrarenal Doppler ultrasound features are combined, the accuracy of color flow Doppler ultrasound in the detection TRAS is reported to be 95%.[16,25]

The gold standard technique in the diagnosis of TRAS is DSA. In patients with renal insufficiency carbon dioxide may be used as a contrast agent in the diagnostic angiographic procedure. Percutaneous transluminal angioplasty (PTA) with or without stent placement is accepted as a first-choice treatment method in TRAS because of its relative low morbidity in comparison to surgical correction. The success rate of PTA was reported as ranging between 85% and 93%.[30] After PTA treatment, normalization of PSV at the stenotic artery and acceleration time with the disappearance of parvus-tardus waveform in the intrarenal artery suggests successful revascularization.[7]

Renal Artery Thrombosis

Renal artery thrombosis (RAT) is the least common vascular complication of vascular transplant with an occurrence rate of less than 1% of all renal transplantations.[31,32] RAT usually results from a technical problem, such as intimal dissection, kinking or torsion of the vessels during organ retrieval, and implantation and discrepancy between the donor and recipient arteries. Predisposing factors of RAT are poor cardiac output, hyperacute rejection, presence of antiphospholipid antibody and cryoglobulins, external compression by adjacent hematoma, and toxicity of immunosupressive agents such as cyclosporine or sirolimus.[32–34] RAT usually occurs in the early postoperative period. Late onset RAT results from renal artery stricture or graft rejection. Kidneys with more than one renal artery are more prone to present with RAT after transplantation.[8] Presenting symptoms include sudden cessation of urine output with severe tubular necrosis and rejection. Color flow Doppler ultrasound demonstrates an absence of flow in the main and intrarenal arteries (**Fig. 4**). Contrast-enhanced CT and MR imaging reveal complete loss of perfusion over the graft kidney. MR angiography can demonstrate the RAT without using intravenous contrast enhancement. Radionuclide imaging demonstrates severe reduction or absence of allograft perfusion. The presence of RAT is an indication for emergency revascularization.

Renal Vein Thrombosis

Renal vein thrombosis (RVT) is a serious condition that may result in graft loss. Reported incidence of RVT is 0.9% to 4.5%.[35] Causes of RVT include compression due to hematomas, hypovolemia, angulation or kinking of the vein, anastomotic strictures, slow flow secondary to rejection or an underlying state of deep venous thrombosis, or hypercoaguability.[36] RVT usually occurs suddenly in the first week following the transplantation. Eighty percent of RVT occurs in the first month.[37] Chronic or partial RVT causes chronic venous

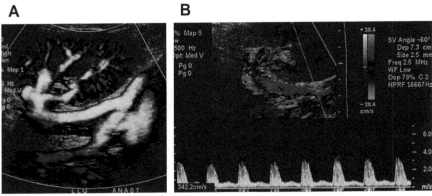

Fig. 2. Transplant renal artery stenosis. (*A*) Power Doppler ultrasound reveals transplant renal vasculature. (*B*) Spectral Doppler ultrasound reveals increased PSV (342.2 cm/s) of transplant renal artery suggesting TRAS.

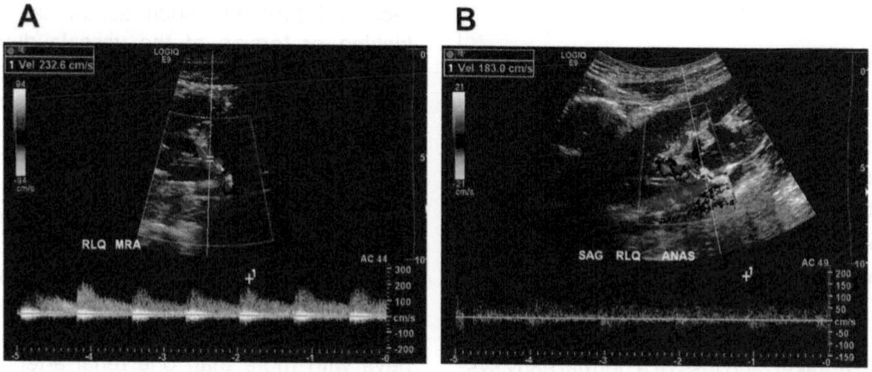

A **B**

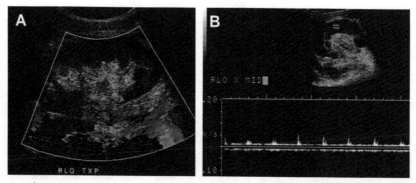

Fig. 3. Increased PSV in the early postoperative period. (*A*) Spectral flow Doppler ultrasound demonstrates increased velocity (232 cm/s) in the transplant renal artery suggesting TRAS. (*B*) Follow-up after 1 day demonstrates renal artery velocity to be 183 cm/s, suggesting that first day increased velocity was secondary to postoperative changes.

hypertension, which may result in the development of peritransplant venous collaterals.[38] Left lower quadrant allografts are more frequently prone to have RVT, attributed to "silent iliac artery compression syndrome," which is described as a compression of the left common iliac vein between the sacrum and the left common iliac artery.[20] Patients present with oliguria, hematuria, graft tenderness, and swelling. Gray-scale ultrasound demonstrates enlarged graft kidney with hypoechoic appearance, loss of cortico-medullary distinction, effacement of renal sinus, and collecting system and an echogenic thrombus within the dilated transplant vein.[15,39] To prevent false negative ultrasound examinations in terms of RVT, routine color flow Doppler ultrasound examination of the renal graft should reveal the patency of the venous anastomosis with an appearance of inverted T shape representing end-to-side anastomosis of the transplanted renal vein to the iliac vein. Color flow Doppler ultrasound demonstrates complete absence of blood flow in the renal vein in the setting of RVT (**Fig. 5**). It should be kept in mind that no venous outflow may also be observed in RAT. Spectral Doppler of the renal artery reveals sharp systolic wave and absent or reversed diastolic flow secondary to increased resistance. RI in intrarenal arteries is markedly elevated in RVT. A low-amplitude tardus–parvus waveform within the intrarenal arteries and transplant renal artery may be observed on spectral Doppler ultrasound.[26,40] Reversal of diastolic flow on spectral Doppler ultrasound may be also encountered in superacute severe rejection, acute tubular necrosis, peritransplant hematoma, vascular kink, and glomerulosclerosis of the renal graft (**Fig. 6**). However, in these situations, reversal of flow is limited to the early diastole, whereas in RVT reversal of flow exists during the entire diastole.[7] Recognition of reversed diastolic flow on spectral Doppler ultrasound is crucial because 33% to 55% of renal grafts with reversed diastolic flow result in dysfunction of the graft.[41–43] Duration of reversed diastolic flow is important for the transplant

Fig. 4. Renal transplant, status post day 1. (*A*) Color flow Doppler demonstrates absence of blood flow within the renal transplant. (*B*) Spectral Doppler image demonstrates transmitted "wall thump" pulsation of an occluded renal artery.

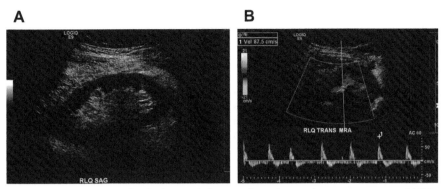

Fig. 5. Renal transplant, status post day 3. Gray-scale image of renal transplant appears normal (*A*) but the color flow Doppler (*B*) demonstrates reversal of diastolic flow suggestive of RVT. Renal vein could not be identified (not shown).

outcome. Reversed diastolic flow present throughout diastole indicates poor outcome of renal transplant.[41–44] In the setting of partial or chronic RVT, reversal of diastolic flow may be absent on spectral Doppler ultrasound secondary to venous flow in peritransplant venous collaterals, which reduce the renal resistance. MR venography may be used to confirm the RVT.

Occurrence time period of reversed diastolic flow is also crucial for transplant outcome. Lockhart and colleagues[45] reported that patients with peritransplant hematoma and vascular kinking can have reversed diastolic flow within the first 24 hours of transplantation and these patients regain graft function after appropriate therapy.

Renal Vein Stenosis

RVS is a rare complication of renal transplant and may result from thrombus formation at the anastomosis site, perivascular fibrosis, or compression from adjacent, large perinephric fluid collections.[46] Detection of RVS is important because RVT may gradually develop from RVS.[47] Color flow Doppler

ultrasound reveals a focal area of aliasing in RVS. Spectral Doppler ultrasound demonstrates high velocity on the stenotic segment. A 3- to 4-fold increase in the PSV in renal vein segment indicates significant stenosis.[48] RVS secondary to partial venous thrombus may cause high RI in the intrarenal arteries.[1] The gold standard imaging technique for the diagnosis of RVS is DSA.

Pseudoaneurysms of the Renal Artery

Estimated prevalance of extrarenal arterial pseudoaneurysm is less than 1% of renal transplant patients.[49] Pseudoaneurysms of renal artery are related to poor surgical technique and perivascular infection. Pseudoaneurysms most frequently occur at the anastomosis site. Rupture of the extrarenal pseudoaneurysms has a high mortality. Most pseudoaneurysms resolve spontaneously. Large (>2 cm in diameter) or progressively enlarged pseudoaneurysms are advised to be treated with intervention.[3]

Gray-scale ultrasound demonstrates an anechoic cystic lesion arising from transplant renal

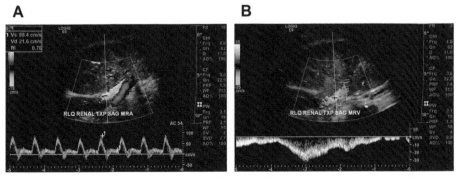

Fig. 6. Acute tubular necrosis. Status post transplant 1 day. (*A*) Color flow Doppler demonstrates reversal of diastolic flow in the main renal artery and (*B*) patent renal vein. On follow-up reversal of diastolic flow disappeared confirming this to be acute tubular necrosis (not shown).

artery with a round or oval shape. Yin-and-yang and to-and-fro signs can be seen with color flow Doppler ultrasound.

Intrarenal Arteriovenous Fistula and Pseudoaneurysm

Intrarenal arteriovenous fistula (AVF) occurs as a complication of renal biopsy with an incidence ranging between 1% and 18%.[50] Simultaneous laceration of both artery and vein results in AVF, whereas pseudoaneurysm occurs when only an arterial branch is lacerated. Gross hematuria is seen in 5% to 7% patients after renal transplant biopsy.[51] Presenting symptoms include hematuria, hypertension, and deterioration of renal function. Large AVFs may cause renal graft ischemia secondary to steal phenomenon. Predisposing factors for AVF include early posttransplant period, the presence of hypertension, sclerosis, and interstitial fibrosis and intrarenal hematoma. Matsell and colleagues[52] reported that about 70% of cases resolve spontaneously within weeks or months.

Color flow Doppler ultrasound is the mainstay imaging technique in the depiction of AVFs (**Fig. 7**A). The AVFs manifest with aliasing from perifistula vibrations on color flow Doppler images. A small color Doppler box with magnification may improve visualization of small intrarenal A-V fistulas and pseudoaneurysms.[7] Spectral Doppler ultrasound reveals a focal area of high-velocity turbulent flow (see **Fig. 7**B). Increasing repetition frequency may distinguish AVF from other vascular flow in the renal parenchyma because the normal renal vasculature loses signal on images acquired with high pulse repetition frequency.[39] Feeding artery manifests with low impedance, high flow velocity, and decreased RI.[46] A draining renal vein may appear as dilated, pulsatile vessels on color flow Doppler ultrasound

secondary to increased intraluminal flow. Spectral Doppler ultrasound reveals arterial waveform in the draining vein.[1]

AVF needs to be treated if bleeding persists more than 72 hours, marked deterioration of renal function, enlarged lesion, and suspicion of steal phenomenon.[1] Angiography detects the size and location of the AVF.[53] Intrarenal pseudoaneurysms present on gray-scale ultrasound as a simple or complex renal cyst with anechoic or hypoechoic appearance (**Fig. 8**A). Color flow Doppler ultrasound reveals yin-and-yang pattern representing vortex of flow (see **Fig. 8**B). Pseudoaneurysms with a narrow neck manifest with to-and-fro waveform in the neck on spectral Doppler ultrasound. Pseudoaneurysms with a broad neck may not exhibit to-and-fro waveform but a turbulent flow with low resistance may be observed on color and spectral Doppler ultrasound, respectively.[46] A simultaneous demonstration of renal artery and vein on MR angiography suggests the presence of AVF.

Renal Artery Kinks

Transplant renal artery kinking may be related to malposition of the graft or restricted space within the transplant bed in the iliac fossa. This kinking occurs when the right kidney with short renal vein and long renal artery is implanted and vascular anastomoses are inappropriately placed.[54] Spectral Doppler ultrasound demonstrates a focal area of increased velocity in the main renal artery, tardus-parvus waveform in the distal intrarenal artery with prolonged acceleration time, and diminished acceleration index. Computed tomography and MR imaging demonstrate the vascular pedicle kinking with multiplanar imaging capability. Angiography reveals kinks of the renal artery and differentiates kinking of the artery from TRAS.

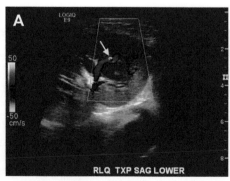 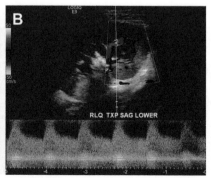

Fig. 7. Arteriovenous fistula in the transplant kidney. (A) Color flow Doppler ultrasound demonstrates AVF (*arrow*) with aliasing in the renal parenchyma. (B) Spectral Doppler ultrasound reveals high-velocity flow with low resistance in the fistula.

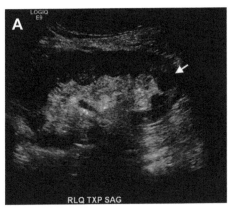
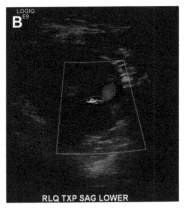

Fig. 8. Pseudoaneurysm in the renal transplant. (A) Gray-scale ultrasound demonstrates an anechoic well-defined cystic lesion (arrow) in the lower pole of the kidney. (B) Color flow Doppler ultrasound reveals yin-yang flow pattern within the pseudoaneurysm.

Allograft Torsion

Improper position of the allograft may result in allograft torsion. In the setting of allograft torsion the kidney rotates around the vascular hilum, resulting in impaired perfusion of the kidney. The discrepancy (>2 cm) between lengths of the renal artery and vein was suggested to be responsible for kinking of the renal pedicle and resulting graft torsion.[55] In allograft torsion ultrasound demonstrates change in the axis of the transplant kidney. Color flow Doppler ultrasound reveals reduced or absent perfusion of the renal parenchyma. The main renal artery segment proximal to the twist presents with increased velocity and reversed diastolic flow on spectral Doppler ultrasound. The distal part of the renal artery has a poststenotic waveform pattern with increased acceleration time. Computed tomography and MR imaging reveal a change in the renal graft orientation and vascular pedicle kinking.

Infarction

Renal graft infarction occurs secondary to occlusion of main and/or intrarenal arteries. Occlusion of intrarenal arteries is more common than of the main renal artery. Small segmental infarcts may be secondary to vasculitis. Segmental infarct of renal transplant appears on gray-scale ultrasound as a poorly marginated hypoechoic area. A diffusely enlarged kidney with hypoechoic appearance on ultrasound suggests global infarction. Color flow and power Doppler ultrasound demonstrates a wedge-shaped area with no vascular flow in focal infarcts (Fig. 9). Dynamic enhanced MR including angiography can reveal both arterial thrombosis and an infarcted segment in the transplant kidney.

Percutaneous angiographic thrombolytic treatment may be helpful in recanalization of the thrombosed segment and reperfusion of the infarcted area. In the setting of diffuse infarction, thrombolytic treatment may result in allograft salvage.

Hematoma

Peritransplant hematomas usually occur in the early postoperative period resulting from small leakage at the vascular anastomosis sites, bleeding from the surface of the renal allograft or from surrounding tissues. Causes of peritransplant hematoma include intraoperative trauma and biopsy but spontaneous hematoma formation may also occur. Hematomas cause symptoms if they are large and cause compression of the neighboring graft parenchyma, vessels, and urinary system. Ultrasound appearances of hematomas are variable. Acute hematomas present with hyperechoic appearance. Over time hematomas become less echogenic. Chronic hematomas with anechoic appearance on ultrasound may mimic other fluid collections such as lymphocele or urinoma. Color flow Doppler ultrasound reveals no vascular flow within the hematomas in the absence of active extravasation. Large

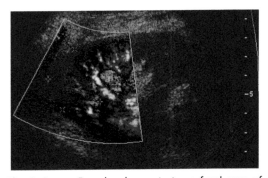

Fig. 9. Power Doppler demonstrates a focal area of infarct (within calipers) in a patient with renal transplant.

hematomas can produce mass effect and result in Page kidney, which presents with hypertension and graft loss.[56]

SUMMARY

Renal transplant provides much longer survival than hemodialysis and peritoneal dialysis for patients with end-stage kidney disease. Prevention of complications in recipients improves survival rates. Imaging studies are crucial for the early recognition of vascular complications of renal transplant. Ultrasound is the key imaging method in the evaluation of renal transplants in the immediate postoperative period and the long-term follow-up. Color flow Doppler ultrasound depicts most vascular complications. Color flow and spectral Doppler ultrasound not only detect and characterize the vascular abnormality in the renal transplant but also can be used for monitoring the outcome of revascularization after surgery or endovascular treatment. Awareness of imaging findings of vascular complications in renal transplant facilitates accurate diagnosis of the complication and prevents graft loss.

REFERENCES

1. Irshad A, Ackerman SJ, Campbell AS, et al. An overview of renal transplantation: current practice and use of ultrasound. Semin Ultrasound CT MR 2009;30(4):298–314.
2. Kocak T, Nane I, Ander H, et al. Urological and surgical complications in 362 consecutive living related donor kidney transplantations. Urol Int 2004;72:252–6.
3. Park SB, Kim JK, Cho KS. Complications of renal transplantation: ultrasonographic evaluation. J Ultrasound Med 2007;26(5):615–33.
4. Akbar SA, Jafri SZ, Amendola MA, et al. Complications of renal transplantation. Radiographics 2005; 25(5):1335–56.
5. Parthipun A, Pilcher J. Renal transplant assessment: sonographic imaging. Ultrasound Clin 2010; 5:379–99.
6. Kok T, Slooff MJ, Thijn CJ, et al. Routine Doppler ultrasound for the detection of clinically unsuspected vascular complications in the early postoperative phase after orthotopic liver transplantation. Transpl Int 1998;11:272–6.
7. Gao J, Ng A, Shih G, et al. Intrarenal color duplex ultrasonography: a window to vascular complications of renal transplants. J Ultrasound Med 2007; 26(10):1403–18.
8. Rajiah P, Lim YY, Taylor P. Renal transplant imaging and complications. Abdom Imaging 2006;31(6): 735–46.
9. Perrella RR, Duerinckx AJ, Tessler FN, et al. Evaluation of renal transplant dysfunction by duplex Doppler sonography: a prospective study and review of the literature. Am J Kidney Dis 1990;15: 544–50.
10. Langer JE, Jones LP. Sonographic evaluation of the renal transplant. Ultrasound Clin 2007;2:73–88.
11. Russo E, Cerbone V, Sciano D, et al. Posttransplant renal monitoring with B-flow ultrasonography. Transplant Proc 2010;42(4):1127–9.
12. Cosgrove DO, Chan KE. Renal transplants: what ultrasound can and cannot do. Ultrasound Q 2008;24(2):77–87.
13. Kim JH, Eun HW, Lee HJ, et al. Clinical use of renal perfusion imaging by means of harmonic sonography with a microbubble contrast agent in patients after renal transplantation: preliminary study. J Ultrasound Med 2005;24:755–62.
14. Sebastià C, Quiroga S, Boyé R, et al. Helical CT in renal transplantation: normal findings and early and late complications. RadioGraphics 2001; 21(5):1103–17.
15. Irshad A, Ackerman S, Sosnouski D, et al. A review of sonographic evaluation of renal transplant complications. Curr Probl Diagn Radiol 2008; 37(2):67–79.
16. Fervenza FC, Lafayette RA, Alfrey EJ, et al. Renal artery stenosis in kidney transplant. Am J Kidney Dis 1998;31(1):142–8.
17. Zerati Filho M, Furtado PS, Barroso U Jr, et al. Kidney transplantation in children: a 50-case experience. Int Braz J Urol 2005;31(6):558–61.
18. Mazzucchi E, Souza AA, Nahas WC, et al. Surgical complications after renal transplantation in grafts with multiple arteries. Int Braz J Urol 2005;31(2): 125–30.
19. Audard V, Matignon M, Hemery F, et al. Risk factors and long-term outcome of transplant renal artery stenosis in adult recipients after treatment by percutaneous transluminal angioplasty. Am J Transplant 2006;6(1):95–9.
20. Jordan ML, Cook GT, Cardella CJ. Ten years of experience with vascular complications in renal transplantation. J Urol 1982;128:689–92.
21. Dimitroulis D, Bokos J, Zavos G, et al. Vascular complications in renal transplantation: a single-center experience in 1367 renal transplantations and review of the literature. Transplant Proc 2009; 41(5):1609–14.
22. Takahashi M, Humke U, Girndt M, et al. Early posttransplantation renal allograft perfusion failure due to dissection: diagnosis and interventional treatment. AJR Am J Roentgenol 2003;180(3): 759–63.
23. Gang S, Rajapurkar M. Vascular complications following renal transplantation. J Nephrol Ren Transplant 2009;2(1):122–32.

24. Sandhu C, Patel U. Renal transplantation dysfunction: the role of interventional radiology. Clin Radiol 2002;57:772–83.

25. de Morais RH, Muglia VF, Mamere AE, et al. Duplex Doppler sonography of transplant renal artery stenosis. J Clin Ultrasound 2003;31(3):135–41.

26. Baxter GM, Ireland H, Moss JG, et al. Colour Doppler ultrasound in renal transplant artery stenosis: which Doppler index? Clin Radiol 1995;50(9):618–22.

27. Patel U, Khaw KK, Hughes NC. Doppler ultrasound for detection of renal transplant artery stenosis-threshold peak systolic velocity needs to be higher in a low-risk or surveillance population. Clin Radiol 2003;58(10):772–7.

28. Thalhammer C, Aschwnden M, Mayr M, et al. Duplex sonography after living donor kidney transplantation: new insights in the early postoperative phase. Ultraschall Med 2006;27(2):141–5.

29. Kim SH. Vascular diseases of the kidney. In: Kim SH, editor. Radiology illustrated: uroradiology. Philadelphia: WB Saunders Co; 2003. p. 429–32.

30. Beecroft JR, Rajan DK, Clark TW, et al. Transplant renal artery stenosis: outcome after percutaneous intervention. J Vasc Interv Radiol 2004;15(2):1407–13.

31. Bakir N, Sluiter WJ, Ploeg RJ. Primary renal graft thrombosis. Nephrol Dial Transplant 1996;11(1):140–7.

32. Irish A. Hypercoagulability in renal transplant recipients. Identifying patients at risk of renal allograft thrombosis and evaluating strategies for prevention. Am J Cardiovasc Drugs 2004;4(3):139–49.

33. Groggel CG. Acute thrombosis of the renal transplant artery: a case report and review of the literature. Clin Nephrol 1991;36(1):42–5.

34. Beyga ZT, Kahan BD. Surgical complications of renal transplantation. J Nephrol 1998;11(3):137–45.

35. Aslam S, Salifu MO, Ghali H, et al. Common iliac artery stenosis presenting as renal allograft dysfunction in two diabetic recipients. Transplantation 2001;71(6):814–7.

36. Penny MJ, Nankivell BJ, Disney AP, et al. Renal graft thrombosis: a survey of 134 consecutive cases. Transplantation 1994;58(5):565–9.

37. Kobayashi K, Censullo ML, Rossman LL, et al. Interventional radiologic management of renal transplant dysfunction: indications, limitations, and technical considerations. Radiographics 2007;27(4):1109–30.

38. McArthur TA, Lockhart ME, Robbin ML. High venous pressure in the main renal vein causing development of peritransplant venous collaterals in renal transplant patients: a rare finding. J Ultrasound Med 2011;30(12):1731–7.

39. Browne RF, Tuite DJ. Imaging of the renal transplant: comparison of MRI with duplex sonography. Abdom Imaging 2006;31(4):461–82.

40. Reuther G, Wanjura D, Bauer H. Acute renal vein thrombosis in renal allografts: detection with duplex Doppler US. Radiology 1989;170(2):557–8.

41. Kaveggia LP, Perrella RR, Grant EG, et al. Duplex Doppler sonography in renal allografts: the significance of reversed flow in diastole. AJR Am J Roentgenol 1990;155:295–8.

42. Mazuecos A, Garcia T, Alonso F, et al. Value of reversed diastolic flow in Doppler sonography of renal transplant. Transplant Proc 1997;29:167–8.

43. Saarinen O, Salmela K, Ahonen J, et al. Reversed diastolic blood flow at duplex Doppler: a sign of poor prognosis in renal transplantation. Acta Radiol 1994;35:10–4.

44. Kribs SW, Rankin RN. Doppler ultrasonography after renal transplantation: value of reversed diastolic flow in diagnosing renal vein obstruction. Can Assoc Radiol J 1993;44:434–8.

45. Lockhart ME, Wells CG, Morgan DE, et al. Reversed diastolic flow in the renal transplant: perioperative implications versus transplants older than 1 month. AJR Am J Roentgenol 2008;190(3):650–5.

46. Brown ED, Chen MY, Wolfman NT, et al. Complications of renal transplantation: evaluation with US and radionuclide imaging. Radiographics 2000;20(3):607–22.

47. Aschwanden M, Thalhammer C, Schaub S, et al. Renal vein thrombosis after renal transplantation: early diagnosis by duplex sonography prevented fatal outcome. Nephrol Dial Transplant 2006;21:825–6.

48. Tublin ME, Dodd GD. Sonography of renal transplantation. Radiol Clin North Am 1995;33:447–59.

49. Bracale UM, Carbone F, del Guercio L, et al. External iliac artery pseudoaneurysm complicating renal transplantation. Interact Cardiovasc Thorac Surg 2009;8(6):654–60.

50. Bach D, Wirth C, Schott G, et al. Percutaneous renal biopsy: 3 years of experience with the biopsy gun in 761 cases—a survey of results and complications. Int Urol Nephrol 1999;31(1):15–22.

51. Boschiero LB, Saggin P, Galante O, et al. Renal needle biopsy of the transplant kidney: vascular and urologic complications. Urol Int 1992;48:130–3.

52. Matsell DG, Jones DP, Boulden TF, et al. Arteriovenous fistula after biopsy of renal transplant kidney: diagnosis and treatment. Pediatr Nephrol 1992;6(6):562–4.

53. Loffroy R, Guiu B, Lambert A, et al. Management of post-biopsy renal allograft arteriovenous fistulas

with selective arterial embolization: immediate and long-term outcomes. Clin Radiol 2008;63(6): 657–65.

54. Miah M, Madaan S, Kessel DJ, et al. Transplant renal artery kinking: a rare cause of early graft dysfunction. Nephrol Dial Transplant 2004;19(7): 1930–1.

55. Smith RB, Ehrlich RM. The surgical complications of renal transplantation. Urol Clin North Am 1976; 3(3):621–46.

56. Sutherland T, Temple F, Chang S, et al. Sonographic evaluation of renal transplant complications. J Med Imaging Radiat Oncol 2010;54(3): 211–8.

Prostate Biopsies and Controversies

Ahmet Tuncay Turgut, MD[a],*, Erkan Kismali, MD[b],
Vikram Dogra, MD[c]

KEYWORDS

• Prostate • Transrectal ultrasound • Biopsy

KEY POINTS

- Transrectal ultrasound (TRUS)-guided prostate biopsy plays a crucial role in the management of prostate cancer.
- A unique feature of the procedure is that it involves zone-based systematic sampling from the regions of the prostate where the tumor is most likely located rather than being lesion directed alone.
- This approach is mainly related to the multicentric nature of the disease and the limited diagnostic ability of TRUS for cancer detection.
- During prostate biopsy, targeted sampling based on TRUS findings cannot preclude the need for systematic sampling, despite currents improvements in the accuracy of cancer detection.
- Periprostatic anesthetic injection is the most effective and commonly preferred method of anesthesia to relieve patient discomfort associated with TRUS-guided biopsy.

DISCUSSION OF PROBLEM/CLINICAL PRESENTATION

Prostate cancer, the most common malignancy and second leading cause of cancer-related death in men, is not only a major medical problem but also a significant public health issue because it may cause significant economic burden.[1] The main diagnostic tools for the disease are digital rectal examination (DRE), serum levels of prostate-specific antigen (PSA), and TRUS-guided biopsy.[2] Among these, TRUS-guided biopsy of the prostate is currently accepted as the gold standard method for diagnosis of prostate cancer.

In clinical practice, the main reason for the referral of patients for TRUS evaluation is guidance for prostate biopsy, although the technique can also be used for the evaluation of the involvement of the prostate gland by various benign and malignant disorders, such as benign prostatic

---

Learning objectives

1. To review the indications for TRUS-guided biopsy of the prostate

2. To reveal the role of imaging tools on the sampling technique in prostate biopsy

3. To evaluate the efficacy of different forms of anesthesia for relieving patient discomfort and/or pain associated with the prostate biopsy

4. To discuss the impact of the number and locations of the biopsy cores on the diagnostic accuracy of transrectal sonographic biopsy of the prostate

---

hyperplasia (BPH), prostatitis, obstructive infertility, and prostate cancer.[3] Contrary to the digitally guided prostate biopsies performed before the ultrasound era, combined use of TRUS and needle biopsy has provided significant increase in the

---

[a] Department of Radiology, Ankara Training and Research Hospital, Ankara 06590, Turkey; [b] Department of Radiology, School of Medicine, University of Ege, Izmir 35100, Turkey; [c] Department of Imaging Sciences, University of Rochester School of Medicine, 601 Elmwood Avenue, Box 648, Rochester, NY 14642, USA
* Corresponding author.
E-mail address: ahmettuncayturgut@yahoo.com

Ultrasound Clin 8 (2013) 605–615
http://dx.doi.org/10.1016/j.cult.2013.07.005
1556-858 13/$ – see front matter © 2013 Elsevier Inc. All rights reserved.

accuracy of diagnosis of prostate cancer by directing the biopsy needle precisely into the target region.

TRUS guidance has dramatically changed with advances in TRUS technology. Today, it is one of the most common outpatient procedures in the urology and radiology practice, with an annual performance of more than 500,000 in the United States.[4] Although there is a broad similarity in practice for various aspects of the procedure, such as indications, preprocedural evalution, sampling technique, and use of anesthesia, there is controversy about several areas.

The main indications for TRUS-guided prostate biopsy are summarized in **Box 1**. DRE, an important component of physical examination in male patients, can identify localized prostate cancer with an irregular shape, hard consistency, and asymmetric shape despite being inherently subjective and having a low accuracy for detection of prostate cancer.[4] Classically, a normal PSA level should be less than 4 ng/mL and a total PSA level exceeding 4 ng/mL is considered to increase the risk for prostate cancer. There is no consensus, however, on the upper limit for normal PSA. Furthermore, low specificity of PSA stands as a significant challenge because its level can be increased not only in prostate cancer but also in benign conditions of prostate, such as BPH and prostatitis.[5] More importantly, prostate neoplasms infrequently are detected in patients with PSA levels in the so-called normal range.[6] In this regard, PSA refinements, such as age-adjusted PSA, PSA velocity, ratio of free PSA/total PSA, and proenzyme (pro) PSA, have been defined for better identification of high-risk individuals who should be referred for biopsy. Age-adjusted PSA levels are not routinely used for screening purposes because of a lack of consensus among practitioners.[6] Accordingly, a PSA velocity value of 0.75 ng/mL or greater per year is considered

suggestive of prostate cancer whereas a PSA density cutoff value of 0.15 was suggested to improve the detection rate of prostate cancer in patients with PSA levels between 4 ng/mL and 10 ng/mL. Another attempt to improve the specificity of PSA screening has been the use of percentage free PSA. Accordingly, it has been shown that a higher rate of cancer detection was noted in patients with a free PSA/total PSA ratio of more than 15%.[7] Pro-PSA, alternatively, is considered better than other forms of PSA to differentiate between cancer and benign conditions in men with PSA values from 2.5 ng/mL to 10 ng/mL.

In some circumstances, TRUS-guided prostate biopsy is contraindicated (**Box 2**).

Preprocedural Evaluation

Patients referred for prostate biopsy should be reassured and informed about the procedure in detail when they arrive in the ultrasound department. Taking into account the potentially high level of patient anxiety, an optimal room setup should be provided to ensure a quiet, warm, and uncrowded environment for the procedure.[8] The preparation of patients for TRUS-guided prostate biopsy is variable among operators. The main steps involved in the preprocedural evaluation of patients undergoing prostate biopsy are given in **Box 3**. First, a written informed consent must be obtained from patients. Although there are no universal guidelines, there has been a consensus on taking measures aimed at preventing infectious complications of the procedure, involving prescribing a bowel cleansing enema and antibiotics before the biopsy. Accordingly, patients are requested to self-administer a bowel-cleansing enema early on the day of the biopsy, although the efficacy of the technique is not strongly supported by some literature data.[9] An additional theoretic benefit for administration of bowel preparations is their potential to improve the quality of TRUS imaging. There are conflicting reports, however, regarding the application and benefit of bowel enema.[9–13] Also, patient

---

Box 1
Indications for TRUS-guided prostate biopsy

Suspicious DRE findings

Elevated levels of serum total PSA

PSA velocity >0.75 ng/mL/y

Free PSA <20%, total PSA in gray zone

Ratio of pro-PSA to free PSA >1.8%

Abnormal TRUS finding(s)

Prior to BPH surgery

Evaluation for recurrence after failed radiation therapy prior to salvage local therapy

---

Box 2
Contraindications for prostate biopsy

Acute prostatitis

Urinary tract infections

Bleeding diathesis

Failure to take antibiotic prophylaxis

Intractable patient anxiety

Acute painful perianal disorders

Box 3
Steps of preprocedural evaluation for prostate biopsy
Informed consent
Questioning of medical history for bleeding diathesis and blood clotting medication
Antibiotic prophylaxis
Rectal enema
Achievement of empty urinary bladder

discomfort after the administration and cost of the agent are suggested as factors against the routine clinical use of bowel preparations before the procedure.

The most commonly recommended practice of antibiotic prophylaxis for TRUS-guided prostate biopsy is ciprofloxacin (Cipro), 500 mg twice daily, beginning before the day of the biopsy and continuing for 3 consecutive days.[5,14] Recently, patients with urethral catheter or diabetes mellitus or those undergoing biopsy with more than 10 cores are reported as prone to urinary tract infection.[15]

Another concern for prostate biopsy is the risk of postprocedural hemorrhage. As an initial precaution, the medical history of patients should be questioned for bleeding diathesis and intake of any medication causing an alteration in blood clotting.[8] Additionally, discontinuation of anticoagulants and nonsteroidal antiinflammatory drugs 7 to 10 days before the biopsy procedure is recommended.[8,16] Nevertheless, discontinuation of low-dose aspirin (<300 mg/d) is not required.[17]

The urinary bladder should not be empty so that a clear interface with the superior margin of the prostate is created, providing a better image quality.

PATIENT DISCOMFORT AND ANESTHESIA

TRUS-guided prostate biopsy, which is routinely performed in an outpatient setting, is a safe and well-tolerated procedure. The procedure, however, is inherently considered uncomfortable because of the size of the ultrasound probe and multiplicity of the cores to be sampled.[16] Several methods of anesthesia have recently been introduced because there has been an increasing concern about patient discomfort during TRUS-guided prostate biopsy. Among these, TRUS-guided periprostatic injection of a local anesthetic agent has proved efficient for increasing patient tolerance during subsequent procedure.[18] The technique involves infiltration of the anesthetic agent (lidocaine without epinephrine) into the prostatoseminal vesical junction where the prostatic plexus provides innervation to the prostate, after the penetration of the Denonvilliers fascia at the posterolateral aspect of the base of the gland by a 22-gauge needle. Consequently, an ultrasound wheal or spreading of the fluid with a hypoechoic appearance filling the white pyramidal site between the prostate and the seminal vesicle laterally is raised, also called a Mount Everest sign because of its white, peaked appearance created by the fat in this location on a sagittal plane (**Fig. 1**).[5] The absence of this finding implies that anesthetic agent might have been injected into the rectal mucosa, resulting in poorer anesthetic effect.[19] Nevertheless, a significant controversy exists regarding the exact site, number, and amount of injections and type of anesthetic agent. The sites of injection described in the literature are the prostatic plexus at the base or apex, prostatic capsule at the apex, and various combinations of these unilaterally or bilaterally.[20–23] The optimal amount of injection for a satisfactory pain control is described as 5 mL to 30 mL,[20,21,24] administered in a total of 1 to 6 injections.[21,22,25] Taking into account the duration of anesthesia, a combination of short-term and long term anesthetics has also

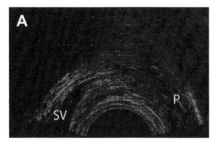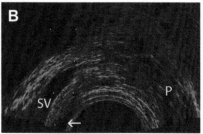

Fig. 1. Sagittal TRUS images before (*A*) and after (*B*) infiltration of the anesthetic agent (lidocaine without epinephrine) into the prostatoseminal vesical junction after the penetration of the Denonvilliers fascia at the posterolateral aspect of the base of the gland by a 22-gauge needle. Spreading of the fluid with a hypoechoic appearance filling the white pyramidal site between the prostate and the seminal vesicle laterally is raised (*arrow* [*B*]), also called the Mount Everest sign. (P, prostate; SV, seminal vesicle.)

been recommended apart from the commonly encountered use of local anesthetics, with shorter duration of effect.[24,26]

The injection of the anesthetic agent is preferably performed in the prebiopsy period to allow sufficient time for effect.[5] Also, it should be kept in mind that the technique might have some potential complications, such as systemic lidocaine toxicity, pain associated with the puncture by the needle used for local anesthesia, the need for repeated local anesthetic injections during the biopsy, distortion or artifact formation on TRUS image, periprostatic infection, and erectile dysfunction.[27,28] The technique has some inherent limitations, however, such as its operator-dependent nature and inefficiency of the technique in the presence of risk factors, such as patient anxiety, young age, repeat biopsies, and inflammatory anal diseases; conscious sedation with intravenous midazolam counteracts these limitations,[29] involving the intravenous injection of midazolam 5 to 10 minutes before biopsy by an anesthetist and noninvasive monitoring during and after the procedure.[4] Another common form of anesthesia for prostate biopsy is administration of lidocaine gel before the procedure,[30] although this method has been reported less efficient than periprostatic anesthetic injection.[20,31]

ANATOMY

The prostate, which is an exocrine gland, is located below the bladder neck and surrounds the urethra. On the superolateral aspect of the gland, the seminal vesicles and the vas deferens lie with a slightly oblique orientation. Anatomically, it is wrapped by a thin pseudocapsule, which can hardly be distinguished from the surrounding fascial planes.[1] On average, 30% of a normal prostate in adulthood consists of the fibromuscular stroma whereas the rest, 70%, is composed of glandular elements.[32] In adults, the dimensions of the normal prostate are 4.0 cm to 4.5 cm, 2.5 cm to 3.0 cm, and 3.0 cm to 4.0 cm in transverse, anteroposterior, and craniocaudal axes, respectively.[1] Conventionally, the glandular prostate is histologically composed of an inner gland (IG), consisting of a transition zone (TZ) and periurethral glandular tissue, and an outer gland, involving a peripheral zone (PZ) and a central zone (CZ). Anatomically, the relative amount of PZ to IG increases from the base of the gland toward the apex.

SONOGRAPHIC ANATOMY

On ultrasound, the appearance of the normal prostate varies depending on age. In young men, the hyperplasia of the glandular tissue is negligible, whereas in older men the development of BPH results in a larger gland with a more rounded shape.[1] Sonographically, IG has a hypoechoic appearance on the anterior aspect of the prostate, whereas the outer PZ is usually homogenous and more echogenic. Importantly, 80% of prostate cancer occurs in PZ, whereas the rest, 20%, develops from CZ. TRUS usually enables the distinction of the hypoechoic transition zone with an anterior location from the echogenic PZ, which is homogenous in echotexture compared with the rest of the gland.[1] In healthy adult men, the CZ can hardly be discerned from PZ on TRUS. The TZ constitutes apparently a larger proportion of the prostate in older men because of associated hyperplastic changes.

IMAGING PROTOCOLS

Mostly, a left lateral decubitis patient position is preferred for TRUS examination because it is well tolerated. Some investigators warn, however, that a lateral decubitis position could increase the color flow Doppler flow in the dependent part of the gland, which potentially causes misinterpretation of the CDUS findings.[32] Usually an accompanying DRE is recommended because it may enable the operator to correlate suspicious physical examination findings with TRUS abnormalities. Today, transrectal scanning of the prostate by biplane probes with a combination of end-viewing and side-viewing transducers involves multiplanar imaging in semicoronal, axial, and sagittal projections. Technically, transducers in the 5 MHz to 8 MHz range provide an optimal resolution for the PZ, which might have a positive impact on the accuracy of the biopsy procedure. Ultrasound gel over a latex condom applied to the probe can help avoid the air artifacts. In a similar fashion, the use of a self-administered enema on the morning of the procedure aids in evacuating gas and feces, which may cause distortion of the TRUS image. Technically, a full urinary bladder providing a clear interface with the prostate base helps in better visualization of the gland. The bladder should not be overdistended, however, because this may cause urinary incontinence during a concomitant prostate biopsy.

TRUS evaluation of the prostate is usually started by systematic scanning in the transverse plane, beginning from the level of seminal vesicles adjacent to the prostate base and continuing down to the apical level with the demonstration of the glandular zones.[8] Then, scanning in the sagittal plane is recommended to confirm any suspicious finding detected in aforementioned planes.

Also, the volume of the prostate can be calculated with the ellipsoid formula by using the diameters in orthogonal axes calculated on TRUS: volume of prostate = $0.52 \times td \times apd \times ccd$, where td, apd, and ccd represent the transverse, anteroposterior, and craniocaudal diameters of the prostate, respectively. In patients with prostate cancer, estimation for prostate volume can be helpful when recommending an appropriate therapy.[8]

IMAGING FINDINGS

On TRUS, a hypoechoic lesion in the PZ can classically represent malignancy, although prostate cancer less frequently has an isoechoic or hyperechoic appearance.[1] Nevertheless, other less-specific imaging features, such as asymmetry of the echotexture or glandular margin, a nonspecific echo irregularity, and a bulge or irregularity in the outline of the capsule, are also helpful for the diagnosis because a significant proportion of prostate cancer is isoechoic.[33] A limitation for the use of gray-scale ultrasound is that approximately half of prostate cancers are invisible by the technique. Moreover, several entities, such as BPH, prostatitis, atrophy, hematoma, ductal ectasia, and prostatic intraepithelial neoplasia, can mimic the gray-scale appearance of prostate cancer, resulting in lower specificity for the diagnosis.[1,34–36]

A challenge for the evaluation of prostate cancer is its mostly multifocal nature, although a solitary focal nodule may appear in 30% of the disease. The lesion is accompanied by an infiltrative component in approximately 50% of patients whereas an infiltrative pattern predominates in the remaining 20%.[35] In advanced disease, diffusely hypoechoic and heterogenous echotexture of the PZ, which is isoechoic or hyperechoic compared with the IG in a normal prostate, is detected (**Fig. 2**). Alternatively, no specific ultrasound feature has been defined for TZ cancers. In patients with concurrent presence of BPH, mixed echo pattern of the entity as well as its compression effect on the PZ, having the potential to mask prostate cancer, may limit the utility of TRUS for evaluation of the prostate.[37] Hence, the value of traditional gray-scale TRUS is limited mainly due to variable tumor echogenecity and lower sensitivity and specificity for cancer detection.[8]

Although color Doppler ultrasound (CDUS) previously was hoped to provide an increase in the diagnosis of prostate cancer, it was later realized that the specificity of the technique for the relevant evaluation was low.[1] Moreover, it was also realized that hypoechoic lesions implying prostate cancer hypervascularity may not necessarily correlate.[8] Nevertheless, color Doppler signal was shown

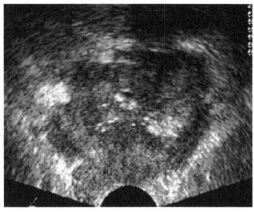

Fig. 2. Prostate cancer. Transverse gray-scale TRUS image demonstrating markedly heterogenous parenchymal echotexture and irregular capsular margins with marked posterior extracapsular extension; the close proximity of the lesion to the rectal wall implies infiltration by cancerous tissue.

highly correlated with stage and the grade of prostate cancer with the post-treatment risk of recurrence. This finding is helpful for the differentiation of low-risk, hypovascular tumors from high-risk, hypervascular tumors because hypervascularity representing a higher rate of Gleason tumor grades and higher risk of extraprostatic spread was typical for the latter group.[38] The technique may have limitations, however, such as the angle dependency of Doppler flow, the intraprostatic noise mimicking increased blood flow, and inadequacy for detecting low flow velocities. Targeted biopsy solely depending, however, on high-frequency color or power Doppler imaging is not recommended, due to the inherent theoretic risk of missing a significant number of cancers.[39]

Power Doppler ultrasound has the advantage of being less angle dependent than CDUS and of detecting slow flow and even minor alterations in blood flow in very small tumoral vessels.[1] The technique was rarely reported, however, as superior to CDUS for the detection of PC.[40] Overall, combined guidance of gray-scale ultrasound and CDUS or power Doppler ultrasound during TRUS-guided biopsy is not sensitive enough to preclude the need for systematic biopsy.[1] Because the increased microvessel density associated with angiogenesis in the cancerous prostate tissue is below the resolution of conventional Doppler imaging, the microbubble contrast agents enabling the visualization of prostatic microvasculature can aid in better detection of prostate cancer.[8]

Contrast-enhanced ultrasound provided a significant improvement for the visualization of prostate cancer by means of the current development of new microbubble-specific ultrasound techniques, enabling better visualization of the microvasculature associated with prostate cancer.[41,42] The sensitivity and specificity of the technique, however, are not still high enough to be able to avoid systematic biopsies.[41] Therefore, the role of contrast-enhanced ultrasound in routine clinical practice is questionable, although targeted sampling incorporated with systematic biopsy protocols increases the detection rate.[41]

Elastography of the prostate involves the evaluation of the elasticity of the prostatic tissue by slight changes in the pressure applied via the probe during TRUS examination, resulting in a change in the real-time ultrasound image constructed, which enables operators to make a distinction between cancerous and benign tissues depending on the hardness gradient and degree of elasticity loss.[33] Although the technique has been considered promising for the detection of prostate cancer, it cannot preclude the requirement for systematic prostate biopsies.[43]

Although TRUS is accepted as the cardinal method for biopsy guidance, its low positive predictive value for the diagnosis of prostate cancer stands as a challenge. Although there has been a consensus regarding the use of TRUS for the assessment of prostate size and for biopsy guidance, its limited value in the early and accurate detection of prostate cancer and the determination of local tumoral extension poses a great clinical challenge for its efficient use. Another limitation for conventional TRUS is that the technique is currently unable to detect high-grade prostatic intraepithelial neoplasia (HGPIN), which is accepted as the most likely precursor lesion to adenocarcinoma of the prostate.

DIAGNOSTIC CRITERIA

Because prostate cancer has a multicentric nature and the diagnostic ability of TRUS alone for cancer detection is limited, TRUS-guided prostate biopsy is based on a zone-based systematic sampling of the regions of the prostate, where the tumors are most likely located. The procedure is performed with biplane transrectal probes, with a combination of end-viewing and/or side-viewing wideband high-frequency transducers (**Fig. 3**). Depending on the technical design of the transducer, the sampling procedure is performed during sagittal or axial scanning. Care should be taken to fire the biopsy gun after indenting the prostate capsule with the biopsy needle, which is necessary to avoid contamination with the periprostatic tissue and enables extraction of a longer tissue sample.[5] Also, operators should predict the extent of the needle trajectory within the gland and

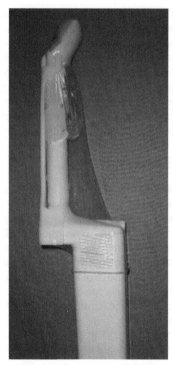

Fig. 3. A stabilizing needle guide is attached to biplane transrectal probe through which a biopsy needle or Chiba needle is passed during the sampling of the prostate and injection of local anesthetic agent.

pay attention to avoid inadvertent penetration of periprostatic tissue and the urethra (**Fig. 4**).[5]

During the procedure, the optimal sites and the number of biopsies have always been an issue of controversy. In general, the procedure involves sampling of the regions of the prostate gland with the highest probability of tumor detection in a spatially oriented fashion.[4] Theoretically, the sampling protocol should involve the PZ because prostate cancer mainly originates from this region

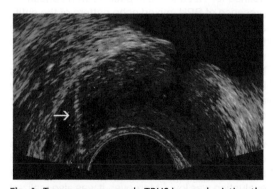

Fig. 4. Transverse gray-scale TRUS image depicting the trajectory of the needle (*arrow*) used for sampling the prostate at midway between the lateral border and the median plane at the level of midgland.

and PZ cancers are more aggressive compared with those originating from the TZ. Nevertheless, routine performance of anterior biopsies involving the sampling of transition zone has also been advocated by some urologists,[44–46] although it is usually recommended in cases with elevated PSA and previous negative biopsies.[47,48] Other urologists, alternatively, have performed midline biopsies,[44,46] although these have been reported to have a lower yield compared with other sampling protocols.[49]

In the early 1980s, TRUS-guided prostate biopsies were first introduced as targeted biopsies for nodular lesions, although later it was realized that they missed a significant number of cancers.[50] The classical sextant sampling sites were the cores at the midway between the lateral border and the median plane at the levels of base, midgland, and apex of the prostate. Several modifications of sextant sampling protocol were introduced, aiming to increase the diagnostic yield with additional cores, particularly from the anatomic regions of the prostate more lateral to the midparasagittal line, decreasing the false-negative outcome of the procedure by sampling

the outer PZ rendering most of the cancers.[51,52] In a study by Eichler and colleagues,[53] sampling protocols with 12 cores, including laterally directed cores and the standard sextant scheme, were reported to provide a balance between the rate of cancer detection and the potential adverse effects of the procedure. The investigators also noted that no significant increase for cancer detection rate was obtained with 18 to 24 core schemes.[53] Currently, extended sampling protocols involving the sampling of 10 to 12 cores are preferred by most practitioners (**Fig. 5**). Other sampling protocols have also been used based on the assumption that an increase in prostate volume has a negative impact on the diagnostic yield, with the number of cores remaining the same.[53,54]

REPEAT BIOPSIES

Abnormal biochemical parameters occasionally persist despite a negative first biopsy. The main indications for repeat prostate biopsies are listed in **Box 4**. Among the indications for a repeat biopsy are a persistently high or rising PSA level (>4 ng/mL), a histopathologic outcome of HGPIN,

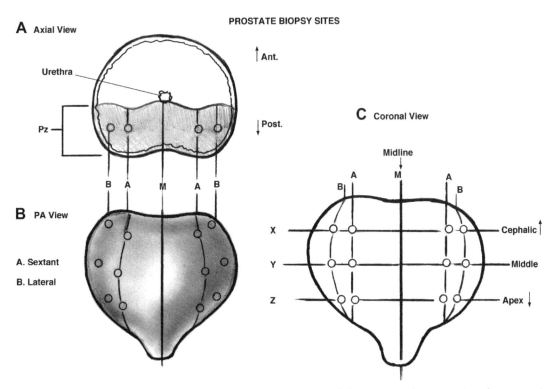

Fig. 5. (A) Axial, (B) posteroanterior (PA), and (C) coronal views of the prostate demonstrating the anatomic localizations of the biopsy cores in sextant (A) and lateral (B) sampling protocols. In the extended sampling protocol, additional cores lateral to the sites for the classical sextant biopsy at the base (X), middle part (Y), and apex (Z) of the prostate are targeted. (From Turgut AT, Dogra VS. Transrectal prostate biopsies. In: Dogra V, Saad W, editors. Ultrasound guided procedures. 1st edition. New York: Thieme; 2009. p. 90; with permission.)

<table>
<tr><td>

Box 4
Indications for repeat prostate biopsy

Persistently elevated or rising PSA level (4 ng/mL)

Suspicious histopathology from the initial biopsy (HGPIN, ASAP, or suspicious but nondiagnostic cellular changes)

Increased prostate volume (>60 mL)

Family history of prostate cancer

PSA velocity >0.75 ng/mL/y

Free PSA/total PSA ratio <0.20

</td></tr>
</table>

or atypical small acinar proliferation (ASAP) from the initial biopsy as well as a previous report of nondiagnostic cellular changes.[4] Technically, areas of the prostate not routinely sampled in the initial biopsy, such as the anterior horn of the PZ and lateral areas, and the IG should be sampled in the repeat biopsy because the initial biopsy may have missed the cancer because of its small volume or its IG location.[1] Also, the number of cores sampled during the procedure should be increased to 24 to decrease the need for a future rebiopsy.[55] In cases of persistent suspicion of prostate cancer despite repeated negative biopsies, however, a saturation biopsy involving the sampling of the gland evenly distributed throughout the gland with 20 or more cores may also be recommended. The latter protocol is based on the assumption that the cancer is too small or located deeply in the gland.[56] An issue of controversy is the time to stop taking repeat biopsies although there is an apparent indication. The likelihood of missing significant prostate cancer has been reported to diminish with each set of repeat biopsies.[57] Accordingly, third and fourth sets of biopsies have not been regarded as mandatory by some investigators.[58,59]

Complications of TRUS-guided biopsy are usually minor, detected in 70% of patients. Among common minor complications are mild urethral bleeding presenting as hematuria or hemospermia, rectal bleeding, infectious complications presenting as acute prostatitis and urinary tact infections, and postprocedural pain or discomfort. Rarely, severe complications, such as severe rectal bleeding or hematuria, prostate infection or abscess causing fever or sepsis, and urinary retention, can be encountered in less than 1% of patients.

PEARLS, PITFALLS, AND VARIANTS

The accuracy of TRUS evaluation of the prostate gland for cancer is not satisfactory.

In the elderly population, evaluation of the prostate by TRUS can be complicated by BPH, which may mask any concurrent cancer because of its mixed echo pattern. Currently, TRUS-guided biopsy with 12 cores is accepted as the gold standard for the diagnosis of prostate cancer in most centers. Imaging data obtained by TRUS cannot preclude the need for systematic sampling of the gland. Although early detection of prostate cancer is critical for a proper management, insignificant cancers as well as significant ones can be detected on histopathologic analysis, which has an impact on patient management. At present, the positive predictive value of prostate biopsies based on DRE, PSA, and TRUS findings is low, resulting in a large number of unnecessary biopsies.

PATHOLOGY

The pathology results for most patients are usually straightforward and definitive, although pathologic analysis of biopsy specimens may infrequently reveal atypical cells consistent with HGPIN.[60] A significant controversy exists for the management of these patients. Mostly, the diagnosis of HGPIN after initial prostate biopsy is regarded as precancerous or concurrent with cancer in a remote location and a repeat prostate biopsy is recommended for patients with relevant histopathology because they are considered to have increased malignancy risk.[8] It is agreed that a repeat biopsy in these patients should involve the sampling of the whole gland, including the IG and high predilection areas of the PZ, rather than focusing on the sites with HGPIN reported in the initial biopsy.[1] Nevertheless, it has also been claimed that immediate repeat biopsy for HGPIN is unnecessary given the low cancer detection rate in repeat biopsy after an initial sampling with 12 cores.[61]

Infrequently, the histopathologic outcome of nondiagnostic cellular changes may be reported after TRUS-guided prostate biopsy. It is considered that insufficiency of the diagnostic material of the previous biopsy is because of the small tumor volume or inappropriate sampling by the needle passing through the edge of an adjacent tumor.[1] Accordingly, a site-specific approach focusing around the suspicious areas is recommended in these patients.

The histopathologic analysis of biopsy specimen also involves the assessment of the biologic potential of the individual tumor, which has a significant impact on patient management. Gleason score, referring to the numeric encoding of the relevant assessment, is a measure of the tumor aggressiveness. It combines discrete primary and secondary patterns or grades into a total of 9 discrete groups (scores 2–10). Accordingly, the primary grade refers to the predominant grade whereas the secondary grade represents the next most common one.

In this regard, a Gleason score of less than 4 is consistent with a well-differentiated cancer whereas a score greater than 7 represents poorly differentiated, aggressive tumors. Apart from the Gleason score, the number of cores harboring the diseased cells and the percentage of tumor in each core are other factors taken into consideration for the management of the tumor and the assessment of the prognosis.

WHAT REFERRING PHYSICIANS NEED TO KNOW

TRUS examination is one of the most reliable tools for referring physicians because it not only enables the evaluation of the sonographic changes associated with various disorders affecting the prostate gland but also provides useful guidance for prostate biopsy. Nevertheless, awareness of the advantages and limitations of the technique is critical, enabling physicians to avoid any mismanagement during the course of the disease.

Currently, it is agreed that TRUS-guided biopsy of the prostate is the gold standard method for diagnosis of prostate cancer. In spite of the similarities between operators in its practice, there is still controversy about several unsettled aspects of the procedure. The procedure is generally safe and well tolerated and may usually be accompanied with minor complications.

SUMMARY

TRUS-guided prostate biopsy plays a crucial role in the management of prostate cancer. A unique feature of the procedure is that it involves zone-based systematic sampling from the regions of the prostate where the tumor is most likely located rather than being lesion directed alone. This approach is mainly related to the multicentric nature of the disease and the limited diagnostic ability of TRUS for cancer detection. Currently, the procedure involves sampling 12 cores from mid-parasagittal and lateral aspects of base, midgland, and apex of the prostate. During prostate biopsy, targeted sampling based on TRUS findings cannot preclude the need for systematic sampling, despite currents improvements in the accuracy of cancer detection. Periprostatic anesthetic injection is the most effective and commonly preferred method of anesthesia to relieve patient discomfort associated with TRUS-guided biopsy.

REFERENCES

1. Turgut AT, Dogra VS. Prostate carcinoma: evaluation using transrectal sonography. In: Hayat MA, editor. Methods of cancer diagnosis, therapy and prognosis. 1st edition. New York: Elsevier; 2008. p. 499–520.
2. Heidenreigh A, Aus G, Bolla M, et al. EAU guidelines on prostate cancer. Eur Urol 2008;53:68–80.
3. Tamsel S, Killi R, Hekimgil M, et al. Transrectal ultrasound in detecting prostate cancer compared with serum total prostate-specific antigen levels. J Med Imaging Radiat Oncol 2008;52:24–8.
4. Turgut AT, Dogra VS. Transrectal prostate biopsies. In: Dogra V, Saad W, editors. Ultrasound guided procedures. 1st edition. New York: Thieme; 2009. p. 85–93.
5. Papatheodorou A, Ellinas P, Tandeles S, et al. Transrectal ultrasonography and ultrasound-guided biopsies of the prostate gland: how, when, and where. Curr Probl Diagn Radiol 2005;34:76–83.
6. Thompson IM, Pauler DK, Goodman PJ, et al. Prevalence of prostate cancer among men with a prostate-specific antigen level <or = 4.0 ng per milliliter. N Engl J Med 2004;350:2239–46.
7. Pelzer AE, Volgger H, Bektic J, et al. The effect of percentage free prostate-specific antigen (PSA) level on the prostate cancer detection rate in a screening population with low PSA levels. BJU Int 2005;96:995–8.
8. Turgut AT, Kismali E, Dogra V. Ultrasound of the prostate: update on current techniques. Ultrasound Clin 2010;5:475–8.
9. Matlaga BR, Eskew LA, McCullough DL. Prostate biopsy: indications and technique. J Urol 2003; 169:12–9.
10. Jeon SS, Woo SH, Hyun JH, et al. Bisacodyl rectal preparation can decrease infectious complications of transrectal ultrasound-guided prostate biopsy. Urology 2003;62:461–6.
11. Zaytoun OM, Vargo EH, Rajan R, et al. Emergence of fluoroquinolone-resistant Escherichia coli as cause of postprostate biopsy infection: implications for prophylaxis and treatment. Urology 2011; 77:1035–41.
12. Carey JM, Korman HJ. Transrectal ultrasound guided biopsy of the prostate. Do enemas decrease clinically significant complications? J Urol 2001;166:82–5.
13. Lindert KA, Kabalin JN, Terris MK. Bacteremia and bacteriuria after transrectal ultrasound guided prostate biopsy. J Urol 2000;164:2145–6.
14. Sadeghi-Nejad H, Simmons M, Dakwar G, et al. Controversies in transrectal ultrasonography and prostate biopsy. Ultrasound Q 2006;22:169–75.
15. Simsir A, Kismali E, Mammadov R, et al. Is it possible to predict sepsis, the most serious

complication in prostate biopsy? Urol Int 2010;84: 395–9.

16. Shandera KC, Thibault GP, Deshon GE Jr. Variability in patient preparation for prostate biopsy among American urologists. Urology 1998;52: 644–6.

17. Maan Z, Cutting CW, Patel U, et al. Morbidity of transrectal ultrasonography-guided prostate biopsies in patients after the continued use of low-dose aspirin. BJU Int 2003;91:798–800.

18. Alavi AS, Soloway MS, Vaidya A, et al. Local anesthesia for ultrasound guided prostate biopsy: a prospective randomized trial comparing 2 methods. J Urol 2001;166:1343–5.

19. Hollingsworth JM, Miller DC, Wei JT. Local anesthesia in transrectal prostate biopsy. Urology 2006;67:1283–4.

20. Nash PA, Bruce JE, Indudhara R, et al. Transrectal ultrasound guided prostatic nerve blockade eases systematic needle biopsy of the prostate. J Urol 1996;155:607–9.

21. Kaver I, Mabjeesh NJ, Matzkin H. Randomized prospective study of periprostatic local anesthesia during transrectal ultrasound-guided prostate biopsy. Urology 2002;59:405–8.

22. Soloway MS, Obek C. Periprostatic local anesthesia before ultrasound guided prostate biopsy. J Urol 2000;163:172–3.

23. Schostak M, Christoph F, Müller M, et al. Optimizing local anesthesia during 10-core biopsy of the prostate. Urology 2002;60:253–7.

24. Ozden E, Yaman O, Göğüs C, et al. The optimum doses of and injection locations for periprostatic nerve blockade for transrectal ultrasound guided biopsy of the prostate: a prospective, randomized, placebo controlled study. J Urol 2003;170:2319–22.

25. Taverna G, Maffezzini M, Benetti A, et al. A single injection of lidocaine as local anesthesia for ultrasound guided needle biopsy of the prostate. J Urol 2002;167:222–3.

26. Lee-Elliott CE, Dundas D, Patel U. Randomized trial of lidocaine vs lidocaine/bupivacaine periprostatic injection on longitudinal pain scores after prostate biopsy. J Urol 2004;171:247–50.

27. Turgut AT, Olcucuoglu E, Kosar P, et al. Complications and limitations related to periprostatic local anesthesia before TRUS-guided prostate biopsy. J Clin Ultrasound 2008;36:67–71.

28. Irani J, Fournier F, Bon D, et al. Patient tolerance of transrectal ultrasound-guided biopsy of the prostate. Br J Urol 1997;79:608–10.

29. Turgut AT, Ergun E, Kosar U, et al. Sedation as an alternative method to lessen patient discomfort due to transrectal ultrasonography-guided prostate biopsy. Eur J Radiol 2006;57:148–53.

30. Issa MM, Bux S, Chun T, et al. A randomized prospective trial of intrarectal lidocaine for pain control during transrectal prostate biopsy: the Emory University experience. J Urol 2000;164:397–9.

31. Seymour H, Perry MJ, Lee-Elliot C, et al. Pain after transrectal ultrasonography-guided prostate biopsy: the advantages of periprostatic local anaesthesia. BJU Int 2001;88:540–4.

32. Halpern EJ, Frauscher F, Strup SE, et al. Prostate: high-frequency Doppler US imaging for cancer detection. Radiology 2002;225:71–7.

33. Loch T. Urologic imaging for localized prostate cancer in 2007. World J Urol 2007;25:121–9.

34. Prando A, Billis A. Focal prostatic atrophy: mimicry of prostatic cancer on TRUS and 3D-MRSI studies. Abdom Imaging 2009;34:271–5.

35. Grossfeld GD, Coakley FV. Benign prostatic hyperplasia: clinical overview and value of diagnostic imaging. Radiol Clin North Am 2000;38:31–47.

36. Tamsel S, Killi R, Ertan Y, et al. A rare case of granulomatous prostatitis caused by mycobacterium tuberculosis. J Clin Ultrasound 2007;35:58–61.

37. Purohit RS, Shinohara K, Meng MV, et al. Imaging clinically localized prostate cancer. Urol Clin North Am 2003;30:279–93.

38. Cornud F, Hamida K, Flam T, et al. Endorectal color doppler sonography and endorectal MR imaging features of nonpalpable prostate cancer: correlation with radical prostatectomy findings. AJR Am J Roentgenol 2000;175:1161–8.

39. Carey BM. Imaging for prostate cancer. Clin Oncol (R Coll Radiol) 2005;17:553–9.

40. Halpern EJ, Sturp SE. Using gray scale and color and power Doppler sonography to detect prostatic cancer. AJR Am J Roentgenol 2000;174:623–7.

41. Wink M, Frauscher F, Cosgrove D, et al. Contrast-enhanced ultrasound and prostate cancer; a multicentre European research coordination project. Eur Urol 2008;54:982–92.

42. Aigner F, Pallwein L, Mitterberger M, et al. Contrast-enhanced ultrasonography using cadence-contrast pulse sequencing technology for targeted biopsy of the prostate. BJU Int 2009;103:458–63.

43. Pallwein L, Mitterberger M, Gradl J, et al. Value of contrast-enhanced ultrasound and elastography in imaging of PC. Curr Opin Urol 2007;17: 39–47.

44. Chen ME, Troncoso P, Johnston DA, et al. Optimization of prostate biopsy strategy using computer based analysis. J Urol 1997;158:2168–75.

45. Terris MK, McNeal JE, Stamey TA. Transrectal ultrasound imaging and ultrasound guided prostate biopsies in the detection of residual carcinoma in clinical stage A carcinoma of the prostate. J Urol 1992;147:864–9.

46. Eskew LA, Bare RL, McCullough DL. Systematic 5 region prostate biopsy is superior to sextant method for diagnosing carcinoma of the prostate. J Urol 1997;157:199–202.

47. Lui PD, Terris MK, McNeal JE, et al. Indications for ultrasound guided transition zone biopsies in the detection of prostate cancer. J Urol 1995;153: 1000–3.
48. Chang JJ, Shinohara K, Hovey RM, et al. Prospective evaluation of systematic sextant transition zone biopsies in large prostates for cancer detection. Urology 1998;52:89–93.
49. Terris MK. Extended field prostate biopsies: too much of a good thing? Urology 2000;55:457–60.
50. Hodge KK, McNeal JE, Terris MK, et al. Random systematic versus directed ultrasound guided transrectal core biopsies of the prostate. J Urol 1989;142:71–4.
51. Presti JC Jr, Chang JJ, Bhargava V, et al. The optimal systematic prostate biopsy scheme should include 8 rather than 6 biopsies: results of a prospective clinical trial. J Urol 2000;163:163–6.
52. Presti JC Jr. Prostate biopsy: how many cores are enough? Urol Oncol 2003;21:135–40.
53. Eichler K, Hempel S, Wilby J, et al. Diagnostic value of systematic biopsy methods in the investigation of PC: a systematic review. J Urol 2006; 175:1605–12.
54. Ozden E, Turgut AT, Talas H, et al. Effect of dimensions and volume of the prostate on cancer detection rate of 12 core prostate biopsy. Int Urol Nephrol 2007;39:525–9.
55. Boczko J, Messing E, Dogra V. Transrectal sonography in prostate evaluation. Radiol Clin North Am 2006;44:679–87.
56. Raja J, Ramachandran N, Munneke G, et al. Current status of transrectal ultrasound-guided prostate biopsy in the diagnosis of prostate cancer. Clin Radiol 2006;61:142–53.
57. Djavan B, Ravery V, Zlotta A, et al. Prospective evaluation of prostate cancer detected on biopsies 1, 2, 3 and 4: when should we stop? J Urol 2001; 166:1679–83.
58. Zlotta AR, Djavan B, Petein M, et al. Prostate specific antigen density of the transition zone for predicting pathological stage of localized prostate cancer in patients with serum prostate specific antigen less than 10 ng/ml. J Urol 1998;160:2089–95.
59. Horninger W, Reissigl A, Klocker H, et al. Improvement of specificity in PSA-based screening by using PSA-transition zone density and percent free PSA in addition to total PSA levels. Prostate 1998; 37:133–7.
60. Bostwick DG, Qian J, Frankel K. The incidence of high grade prostatic intraepithelial neoplasia in needle biopsies. J Urol 1995;154:1791–4.
61. Lefkowitz GK, Sidhu GS, Torre P, et al. Is repeat prostate biopsy for high-grade prostatic intraepithelial neoplasia necessary after routine 12-core sampling? Urology 2001;58:999–1003.

Index

Note: Page numbers of article titles are in **boldface** type.

A

Abscess
    epididymal, 535
    postvasectomy, 547
    scrotal wall, 537
    testicular, 519
Acoustic radiation force impulse-shear wave speed
    elastography, of kidney, 553–556, 559, 562
Acute scrotum, **531–544**
    appendageal torsion, 534
    definition of, 531
    epididymal torsion, 541
    epididymo-orchitis, 519–520, 534–536
    Fournier gangrene, 537–538
    intratesticular abscess, 519
    mumps orchitis, 537
    nonscrotal causes of, 542
    orchitis, 519–520, 537
    Schönlein-Henoch purpura, 540
    scrotal edema, 540
    scrotal hernia, 540
    scrotal wall infections, 537
    segmental testicular infarction, 518–519, 538–540
    spermatic cord torsion in, 516–518, 528
    spontaneous intratesticular hemorrhage, 540–541
    tension hydrocele, 541–542
    testicular torsion, 516–518, 528, 531–534
    venous infarction, 519
Adenomatoid tumors
    extratesticular, 521
    testicular, 514
Allograft torsion, in kidney transplantation, 601
Anesthesia, for prostate biopsy, 607–608
Angiomyolipomas, of kidney, 567, 570, 572–573, 584
Anisotropy, in kidney elastography, 556–557
Antibiotics, for prostate biopsy, 607
Appendageal torsion, 534
Arteriovenous fistulas, in kidney transplantation, 600

B

"Bell-clapper" deformity, in testicular torsion, 517
Biopsy
    kidney, 578
    prostate, **605–615**
Bleeding. *See* Hemorrhage.
Blue dot sign, in appendageal torsion, 534
Bosniak classification, of renal cysts, 568

C

Calcification, of epidermoid cysts, 515
Carcinomas, testicular, 511
Cellulitis
    postvasectomy, 547
    scrotal wall, 537
Chemotherapy, for renal cell carcinoma, 587–589
Choriocarcinomas, testicular, 512–513
Color Doppler evaluation
    for appendageal torsion, 534
    for epididymo-orchitis, 519–520, 534–536
    for Fournier gangrene, 538
    for kidney transplantation, 594, 596–601
    for mumps orchitis, 537
    for penetrating testicular trauma, 529–530
    for prostate lesions, 609
    for scrotal edema, 540
    for scrotal hernia, 540
    for testicular fracture, 528
    for testicular infarction, 518–519, 539–540
    for testicular rupture, 528
    for testicular torsion, 518, 528, 533
    for testicular tumors, 511
        Leydig cell, 514
        lymphomas, 514
        seminomas, 512
        Sertoli cell, 514
Column of Bertin, 583
Computed tomography
    for kidney masses, 583–584
    for kidney transplantation, 595
Contrast enhanced ultrasonography, **509–523**
    contrast agents for, 510–511
    for acute scrotum, 516–520
    for extratesticular lesions, 521
    for kidney masses, **581–592**
        anatomic considerations in, 582–583
        contrast agents for, 581–582
        for ablation monitoring, 586–587
        for angiosuppressive therapy monitoring, 587–589
        for characterization, 582–586
        for fusion imaging, 589–590
        intraoperative, 590
        safety of, 590
    for kidney transplantation, 594
    for prostate lesions, 609–610
    for testicular masses, 511–516
    for testicular trauma, 520–521

Ultrasound Clin 8 (2013) 617–620
http://dx.doi.org/10.1016/S1556-858X(13)00094-7

Index

Contrast (*continued*)
  vascular anatomy for, 510
Cyst(s)
  epidermal, 515–516
  epididymal, 549
  renal, 568, 583–584
  testicular, 516, 549

D

Digital subtraction angiography, for kidney
  transplantation, 595–596
Doppler evaluation. *See also* Color Doppler
  evaluation; Power Doppler evaluation.
  for kidney masses, 577–578
Dynamic elastography, of kidney, 553–554

E

Elastography
  of kidney, **551–564**
    acoustic radiation force impulse-shear wave
      speed, 553–554
    characteristics impact on, 555–557
    fibroscan-transient, 553–554
    normal values in, 557–560
    quasi-static, 552–553
    sampling in, 554–555
    supersonic shear wave imaging, 553–554
    techniques for, 552–554
  of prostate lesions, 610
Embryonal cell carcinomas, testicular, 512–513
End-stage kidney disease, masses in, 575, 577–578
Epidermal cysts, 515–516, 521
Epididymal cysts, postvasectomy, 549
Epididymis
  fracture of, 527
  torsion of, 541
  tubular ectasia of, 547–548
Epididymitis, 527
Epididymo-orchitis, 519–520, 534–536

F

Fibrosarcomas, testicular, 514
Fibroscan-transient elastography, of kidney, 553–554,
  562
Fibrosis, kidney elastography for, 560–563
Foreign bodies, scrotal, 529–530
Fournier gangrene, 537–538
Fractures
  epididymal, 527
  testicular, 528
Fusion imaging, for kidney masses, 589–590

G

Gangrene, Fournier, 537–538
Genitourinary disorders
  acute scrotum, 516–519, **531–544**
  postvasectomy, **545–550**
  prostate biopsies, **605-615**
  renal. *See* Kidney disorders.
  testicular. *See* Testicular disorders.
Germ-cell tumors, testicular, 511–514
Granulomas, sperm, postvasectomy, 548–549

H

Hematoceles, 526–527, 547
Hematomas
  in kidney transplantation, 601–602
  postvasectomy, 546–547
  scrotal wall, 527
  spermatic cord, 527–528
  testicular, 528–529
Hemorrhage
  in prostate biopsy, 607
  postvasectomy, 546–547
  testicular, 540–541
Hernia, scrotal, 540
Hydroceles
  postvasectomy, 549
  tension, 541–542

I

Immunosuppressive therapy, for renal cell
  carcinoma, 587–589
Infarction
  in kidney transplantation, 601
  testicular, 518–519, 538–540
Infections, scrotal wall, 537

K

Kaposi sarcomas, testicular, 514
Kidney disorders
  elastography for, **551–564**
  fibrosis, 560–563
  in transplantation, **593–604**
  masses, 563, **565–579, 581–592**
    angiosuppressive therapy for, 587–589
    biopsy of, 578
    characterization of, 566–575
    contrast methods for, **581–592**
    cystic, 583–584
    detection of, 566
    differential diagnosis of, 572–573
    fusion imaging for, 589–590
    histology of, 573, 575–576
    in end-stage renal disease, 575, 577–578
    intraoperative evaluation of, 590
    percutaneous ablation for, 586–587
    pseudotumors, 583
    safety issues with, 590

solid, 583–586
tumors, 563

L

Leiomyomas, testicular, 514
Leiomyosarcomas, testicular, 514
Leukemia, testicular, 515
Leydig cell tumors, testicular, 514
Lymphomas
    kidney, 570–571
    testicular, 515

M

Mach cone, in kidney elastography, 554
Magnetic resonance imaging, for kidney
    transplantation, 595
Mesenchymal tumors, testicular, 514
Metastasis, to kidney, 570
Microbubbles, as contrast agents, 510–511, 581–590
Mumps orchitis, 537

N

Necrotizing fasciitis, scrotal, 537–540
Nephrectomy, for kidney masses, 590
Nonseminomatous germ-cell tumors, testicular,
    512–514
Nuclear imaging, for kidney transplantation, 595

O

"Onion-ring" appearance, of epidermoid cysts, 515
Orchitis, 519–520, 534–536
    mumps, 537
Osteosarcomas, testicular, 514

P

Pain, postvasectomy, 549
Power Doppler evaluation
    for kidney transplantation, 594
    for prostate lesions, 609
Prostate biopsy, **605–615**
    anatomy of, 608
    anesthesia for, 607–608
    clinical presentation and, 605–607
    diagnostic criteria and, 610–611
    discomfort in, 607–608
    findings in, 609–610
    imaging protocols for, 608–609
    indications for, 606
    pathology in, 612–613
    patient preparation for, 606–607
    pitfalls in, 612
    repeat, 611–612
Pseudoaneurysms

renal artery, 599–600
    testicular, 529
Pseudotumors, kidney, 583
Pyoceles, 535

Q

Quasi-static elastography, of kidney, 552–553

R

Radionuclide imaging, for kidney transplantation, 595
RECIST trial, 587–589
Renal artery, kidney transplantation complications of
    kinks, 600
    pseudoaneurysm, 599–600
    stenosis, 596–597
    thrombosis, 597
Renal cell carcinomas
    biopsy of, 578
    characterization of, 568–570
    cystic, 568–569
    detection of, 566
    differential diagnosis of, 566–568
    elastography for, 564
    histology of, 573–576
    treatment of, 587–589
    versus angiomyolipomas, 567, 570, 572–573, 584
Renal vein, complications of, in kidney
    transplantation, 597–599
Rhabdomyosarcomas
    extratesticular, 521
    testicular, 514
Rupture, testicular, 528–529

S

Sarcomas
    kidney, 570
    testicular, 514
Schönlein-Henoch purpura, 540
Scrotal edema, 540
Scrotal wall
    hematoma of, 527
    infections of, 537
Segmental testicular infarction, 518–519, 538–540
Seminomas, testicular, 512
Sertoli cell tumors, testicular, 514
Sex cord-stromal tumors, testicular, 514
Shear elasticity probe (fibroscan-transient
    elastography), of kidney, 553–554
Shear waves, in kidney elastography, 553–555, 559,
    562
Silent iliac artery compression syndrome, in kidney
    transplantation, 598
Spectral Doppler evaluation
    for kidney masses, 568

Spectral (*continued*)
    for kidney transplantation, 596, 598
    for testicular pseudoaneurysm, 529
Sperm granulomas, postvasectomy, 548–549
Spermatic cord
    hematomas of, 527–528
    torsion of, 516–518, 528, 531–534
Spermatoceles, postvasectomy, 548
Spontaneous intratesticular hemorrhage, 540–541
Stenosis, in kidney transplantation
    renal artery, 596–597
    renal vein, 599
Sunitinib, for renal cell carcinoma, 589
Supersonic shear wave imaging elastography, of
    kidney, 553–554

T

Tension hydrocele, 541–542
Teratomas, testicular, 512–514
Testicular disorders
    abscess, 519
    anatomy of, 525–526
    cysts, 516, 549
    dislocation, 529
    fracture, 528
    hematoma, 528–529
    infarction, 518–519, 538–540
    masses, 511–516
    orchitis, 519–520
    pseudoaneurysm, 529
    rupture, 528
    torsion, 516–518, 528, 531–534
    traumatic, 520–521, **525–530**
    ultrasonographic technique for, 526
    venous infarction, 519
Thrombosis, in kidney transplantation
    renal artery, 597

renal vein, 597–599
Torsion
    allograft, in kidney transplantation, 601
    epididymal, 541
    spermatic cord, 516–518, 528, 531–534
    testicular, 516–518, 528, 531–534
Transplantation, kidney, **593–604**
    anatomic considerations in, 593–594
    elastography for, 561–563
    imaging techniques for, 594–596
    vascular complications of, 596–602
Transrectal ultrasound-guided prostate biopsy,
    605–615
Trauma, testicular, 520–521, **525–530**
Tubular ectasia
    postvasectomy, 547–548
    testicular, 516
Tumors
    kidney. *See* Kidney disorders, masses.
    testicular, 511–516

V

Varicocele, postvasectomy, 549
Vasectomy, **545–550**
    description of, 545
    postoperative complications and changes of,
        546–549
    techniques for, 545–546
Venous infarction, testicular, 519

W

"Whirlpool sign," in testicular torsion, 518, 532

Y

Young's modulus, in kidney elastography, 552–553

United States Postal Service

Statement of Ownership, Management, and Circulation
(All Periodicals Publications Except Requestor Publications)

1. Publication Title	2. Publication Number	3. Filing Date
Ultrasound Clinics	0 0 0 - 7 1 1	9/14/13

4. Issue Frequency	5. Number of Issues Published Annually	6. Annual Subscription Price
Jan/Apr/Jul/Oct	4	$258.00

7. Complete Mailing Address of Known Office of Publication (Not printer) (Street, city, county, state, and ZIP+4®)

Elsevier Inc.
360 Park Avenue South
New York, NY 10010-1710

Contact Person
Stephen Bushing
Telephone (include area code)
215-239-3688

8. Complete Mailing Address of Headquarters or General Business Office of Publisher (Not printer)

Elsevier Inc., 360 Park Avenue South, New York, NY 10010-1710

9. Full Names and Complete Mailing Addresses of Publisher, Editor, and Managing Editor (Do not leave blank)

Publisher (Name and complete mailing address)

Linda Belfus, Elsevier, Inc., 1600 John F. Kennedy Blvd. Suite 1800, Philadelphia, PA 19103-2899

Editor (Name and complete mailing address)

Donald Mumford, Elsevier, Inc., 1600 John F. Kennedy Blvd. Suite 1800, Philadelphia, PA 19103-2899

Managing Editor (Name and complete mailing address)

Adrianne Brigido, Elsevier, Inc., 1600 John F. Kennedy Blvd. Suite 1800, Philadelphia, PA 19103-2899

10. Owner (Do not leave blank. If the publication is owned by a corporation, give the name and address of the corporation immediately followed by the names and addresses of all stockholders owning or holding 1 percent or more of the total amount of stock. If not owned by a corporation, give the names and addresses of the individual owners. If owned by a partnership or other unincorporated firm, give its name and address as well as those of each individual owner. If the publication is published by a nonprofit organization, give its name and address.)

Full Name	Complete Mailing Address
Wholly owned subsidiary of	1600 John F. Kennedy Blvd., Ste. 1800
Reed/Elsevier, US holdings	Philadelphia, PA 19103-2899

11. Known Bondholders, Mortgagees, and Other Security Holders Owning or Holding 1 Percent or More of Total Amount of Bonds, Mortgages, or Other Securities. If none, check box ☐ None

Full Name	Complete Mailing Address
N/A	

12. Tax Status (For completion by nonprofit organizations authorized to mail at nonprofit rates) (Check one)
The purpose, function, and nonprofit status of this organization and the exempt status for federal income tax purposes:
☐ Has Not Changed During Preceding 12 Months
☐ Has Changed During Preceding 12 Months (Publisher must submit explanation of change with this statement)

PS Form 3526, September 2007 (Page 1 of 3 (Instructions Page 3)) PSN 7530-01-000-9931 PRIVACY NOTICE: See our Privacy policy in www.usps.com

---

13. Publication Title	14. Issue Date for Circulation Data Below
Ultrasound Clinics	July 2013

15. Extent and Nature of Circulation			14. Average No. Copies Each Issue During Preceding 12 Months	No. Copies of Single Issue Published Nearest to Filing Date
a. Total Number of Copies (Net press run)			343	350
b. Paid Circulation (By Mail and Outside the Mail)	(1)	Mailed Outside-County Paid Subscriptions Stated on PS Form 3541. (Include paid distribution above nominal rate, advertiser's proof copies, and exchange copies)	151	133
	(2)	Mailed In-County Paid Subscriptions Stated on PS Form 3541 (Include paid distribution above nominal rate, advertiser's proof copies, and exchange copies)		
	(3)	Paid Distribution Outside the Mails Including Sales Through Dealers and Carriers, Street Vendors, Counter Sales, and Other Paid Distribution Outside USPS®	43	62
	(4)	Paid Distribution by Other Classes Mailed Through the USPS (e.g. First-Class Mail®)		
c. Total Paid Distribution (Sum of 15b (1), (2), (3), and (4))			194	195
d. Free or Nominal Rate Distribution (By Mail and Outside the Mail)	(1)	Free or Nominal Rate Outside-County Copies Included on PS Form 3541	55	55
	(2)	Free or Nominal Rate In-County Copies Included on PS Form 3541		
	(3)	Free or Nominal Rate Copies Mailed at Other Classes Through the USPS (e.g. First-Class Mail)		
	(4)	Free or Nominal Rate Distribution Outside the Mail (Carriers or other means)		
e. Total Free or Nominal Rate Distribution (Sum of 15d (1), (2), (3) and (4))			55	55
f. Total Distribution (Sum of 15c and 15e)			249	250
g. Copies not Distributed (See Instructions to publishers #4 (page #3))			94	100
h. Total (Sum of 15f and g)			343	350
i. Percent Paid (15c divided by 15f times 100)			77.91%	78.00%

16. Publication of Statement of Ownership
☐ If the publication is a general publication, publication of this statement is required. Will be printed ☐ Publication not required
in the October 2013 issue of this publication.

17. Signature and Title of Editor, Publisher, Business Manager, or Owner

Stephen R. Bushing – Inventory/Distribution Coordinator

Date
September 14, 2013

I certify that all information furnished on this form is true and complete. I understand that anyone who furnishes false or misleading information on this form or who omits material or information requested on the form may be subject to criminal sanctions (including fines and imprisonment) and/or civil sanctions (including civil penalties).

PS Form 3526, September 2007 (Page 2 of 3)

Moving?

Make sure your subscription moves with you!

To notify us of your new address, find your **Clinics Account Number** (located on your mailing label above your name), and contact customer service at:

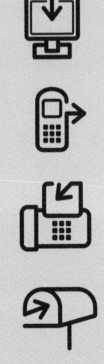

Email: journalscustomerservice-usa@elsevier.com

800-654-2452 (subscribers in the U.S. & Canada)
314-447-8871 (subscribers outside of the U.S. & Canada)

Fax number: 314-447-8029

Elsevier Health Sciences Division
Subscription Customer Service
3251 Riverport Lane
Maryland Heights, MO 63043

ELSEVIER

Printed and bound by CPI Group (UK) Ltd, Croydon, CR0 4YY

03/10/2024

01040378-0009